中医密码

——医之源

Code to Traditional Chinese Medicine

张健君　编著

学苑出版社

图书在版编目（CIP）数据

中医密码：医之源/张健君编著．—北京：学苑出版社，2018.2
（2018.8 重印）

ISBN 978－7－5077－5275－5

Ⅰ.①中…　Ⅱ.①张…　Ⅲ.①中医学　Ⅳ.①R2

中国版本图书馆 CIP 数据核字（2017）第 176808 号

责任编辑：黄小龙
出版发行：学苑出版社
社　　　址：北京市丰台区南方庄 2 号院 1 号楼
邮政编码：100079
网　　　址：www.book001.com
电子邮箱：xueyuanpress@163.com
销售电话：010－67601101（销售部）67603091（总编室）
印　刷　厂：北京画中画印刷有限公司
开本尺寸：787×1092　1/16
印　　　张：13.125
字　　数：215 千字
版　　次：2018 年 2 月第 1 版
印　　次：2018 年 8 月第 2 次印刷
定　　价：66.00 元

秦　序

　　受命撰写该书的序言，实乃诚惶诚恐。历来专著的序言都是由该领域的大家所为，而我非"学院派"中医大夫，更非中医的民间高手。我只是自然科学领域一名普通的研究人员。然而，本书作者张健君大夫的一席话，"中医不是一个行业分类，是一种与生命相关的智慧和践行方法，每个人都该了解。一个局外人看中医，你又是科学家，所以你写本书的序会很有意义"，于我甚是鼓舞。遂受命撰序。

　　作为中国人，通常对中医并不陌生。无论是其阴阳五行基础理论还是针灸、推拿、草药治病，甚至祝由术等，从小到大大家都耳濡目染，略知一二。尽管不是精通其中的道理与逻辑，但大家都能接受中医养生与治病的观点。如同两千多年来的儒、释、道思想一样，中医已融入到每位中国人的血液中。然而，西医自从100多年前进入中国，迅速蓬勃发展，在中国形成了中医和西医并存的局面。遗憾的是，中医并没有得到应有的发展。究其原因，一方面是源于中医师对中医理论基础——《黄帝内经》的理解不同，甚至有歧义，导致了治疗方案上无法形成统一的标准，从而不符合西医标准化治疗的方法，致使中医在国际上无法流行。另一方面，60多年前中国提出了"中西医相结合"的观点，直接导致了现在的中医师在治疗过程中过度依赖西医检查设备来诊断疾病，中医西化现象越来越严重，慢慢偏离了中医的本质，在治疗效果上也不尽人意。于是乎，很多西医师对中医不屑一顾，甚至认为西医是科学的，而中医是非科学的。关于中西医对疾病治疗的争论一直不绝于耳，也没有最终的结论。

　　中医就应该被西医取代而消亡吗？当然不是。中西医有着不同的理论基础。西医是建立在数学、物理和生物学等自然学科和现代解剖学理论基础上，在一些突发性疾病的手术治疗上表现出强大的优势，如血管支架介入治疗急性心肌梗塞，车祸后的手术治疗等等。但是，西医在方法论上采用机械还原论，忽视了生命是一个独立个体的整体特征，是一个非常精妙的系统，直接导致了西医重局部轻整体、重分析轻综合、重物质轻精神等局限性。而中医是建立在道家《易经》的阴阳五行理论基础上的，《黄帝内经》是其理论要典，《伤寒论》和《本草纲目》等是治疗技术要典。中医是天人合一系统论指导下的理论与技术体系，常言的"人体小宇宙，宇宙大人体"可以略窥一斑。故，中西医学对生命认知的理论基础完全不同，相互之间没有兼容性。显然，用西医的理论与观点解释中医的疗效是行不通，而中医的发展用西医来指导更是错误的。所以，"中西医相结合"的观点是值得商榷和反思的。

本人认为，在医学领域，中医的发展无需西医的解释。事实证明，很多西医无法解决的问题，中医却能游刃有余，取得了令人瞩目的神奇疗效。例如，高血压是目前人类的常见疾病之一，西医治疗直接采用各种降压药，而且往往需终身服药。然而，从中医的观点分析，一个人的血压升高是人体某个部位发生问题后人体做出的本能修复反应，治疗之前必须找到病症部位及产生原因，然后才能对症治疗。我本人在一年前突发高血压，如果采用西医治疗，可能需要终身服用降压药。但是，中医师建议我用山楂、冰糖、乌梅加水熬制服用。没有想到，半个月后血压恢复正常，至今也没有反复。再如，糖尿病也是当代常见病之一。一位60多岁的老翁患糖尿病15年，经过西医的多种治疗越来越严重，并表现出严重的并发症，下肢静脉栓塞，几乎失去行动能力。在经过张健君大夫一年多的中药治疗后，现已康复。慢性肾病也是一种常见病之一，到了肾功能衰竭阶段西医治疗方案往往是透析，严重者需要换肾，但是治愈的比率很低。为了进一步证明中医治疗疾病的有效性与高效率，2016年，张健君大夫在全国范围内征集了20名慢性肾病患者。1名患者面诊时因肾脏萎缩，张大夫表示没有康复可能而弃治；1名患者治疗一个月后没有明显好转迹象；其余18名患者停用包括激素在内的所有西药后，经过三个月的纯中医治疗，或恢复正常或维持临床治愈标准已超过一年。尽管这个样本量很小，但是已经足以证明中医的神奇疗效。

张健君大夫是我认识的为数极少的优秀中医师之一。他本人接受的是正宗的西医外科教育，在南京医药大学毕业后从事临床外科手术十余年。然而，在面对无数患者的痛苦和认知西医的局限性之后，他毅然放弃了西医，改学中医，认为中医才是解决人类疾病的终极方案。经过多次的交流，我总结了他对中医的几个观点：（1）中医治疗疾病，并非是人们所认知的中医治疗慢性病，疗效慢，中医治疗只要认知病症成因准确，可以做到立竿见影；（2）中医治疗基于系统论，强调人体的阴阳平衡和经络通畅。所以，一名优秀的中医师，应该可以治愈各种疾病而不是专治某种疾病，因为每种疾病都是人体的阴阳失衡和局部经络堵塞的结果；（3）中药治疗，通常情况下，如果每副药中超过10味药材，这个方子可以基本判断有问题，而且一般不需要使用昂贵的中药材；（4）《黄帝内经》是中医之根本，由于两千多年来文字的演化，我们已经偏离了对《黄帝内经》的正确理解。所以，要想正确还原黄帝与岐伯的对话内涵，需要我们潜心研究每一个汉字的起源与当初的含义。为此，他依然走在潜心研究《黄帝内经》及相关汉字的路上。

《中医密码——医之源》是张健君大夫的第一部作品，它更象是一部介绍中医的科普作品。以通俗的语言，阐明了人体健康与天地运行的关系，详细介绍了阴阳五行和四时六气的中医基本理论模型，及他自己对疾病的认知以及平素养生等重要观点。在本书中还结合一种中药——陈皮来举例说明，一种中药材的功效与产地、种植条件、天时等众多因素之间的关联，以及对不同疾病治疗适应性。全书概念清晰、逻辑缜密、类比恰当，作为外行的我，看后也受益匪浅。本书尽管是中医的科普作品，但是到处体现出了张大夫自己对中医的独特见解，例如，把人体和宇宙回归到能量与信息两个基本单元等，这些对提升我们对中医的正确认知有明显的积极作用。期待也相信本书的出版，会有利于推动中医的发展回到正确的轨道上。

秦高梧　教授，院长

东北大学材料科学与工程学院

2017 年 6 月 1 日

Qin's preface

I was invited to write the preface of this book authored by Doctor Jianjun Zhang, but with profound respect and humility. As well known, the preface of one monograph is usually written by a famous expert in its field, but I am neither an academism doctor of traditional Chinese medicine (TCM), nor a folk expert. I'm just an ordinary researcher in the field of natural science. However, what Doctor Zhang said completely inspired me, "TCM is not one of professional classifications, but is wisdom and practice related to longevity and health, and everyone should understand it and perform it in his daily life. You are a scientist in the field of natural science, as well as an outsider of TCM, and it would be very meaningful if you can write this preface to give your opinions." Accordingly I accepted this invitation to write the preface.

Generally speaking, one Chinese is not unfamiliar with TCM. Most Chinese know it more or less on TCM during their experience of growth, Such as basic theories on the *Yin Yang* and the *Five Phases*, and TCM treatments by acupuncture, massage and herbal remedies, even witch praying. Although we do not understand well the principles and logics of TCM, we usually accept that TCM can preserve health and cure disease. Just like that the ideologies of Confucianism, Buddhism and Taoism spreading more than two thousand years in China, TCM has been integrated into the blood of every Chinese. However, since entered into China more than 100 years ago, Western Medicine (WM) has developed rapidly. A situation of coexistence of TCM and WM in China has formed. Unfortunately, TCM has not been developed that much. One of main reasons is due to the fact that many doctors of TCM have different understandings, even ambiguity, on basic theory of TCM—*Yellow Emperor's Classic of Medicine*. It results in the failure to form unified standards in the treatment of diseases, and that does not conform to the standardized treatment of WM, which makes TCM unable to be popular in the world. The other reason arose from the policy of *Integration between TCM and WM* proposed by Chinese government about 60 years ago. This policy led directly to over – reliance on inspection equipments in the course of diagnose rather than on TCM itself, and more serious westernization of TCM. Finally TCM gradually deviates from the essence itself, and the curative effect is also unsatisfactory. As a result, many WM doctors have a contemptuous disregard on TCM, and they generally consider WM is science while TCM is not. There have been a lot of debates about the treatment of diseases by TCM and WM, but still no solid conclusions.

Should TCM be replaced by WM and die naturally? Certainly not. TCM and WM have different theoretical principles. WM is based on the natural sciences such as mathematics, physics and biology, and modern anatomical theories, etc. It has great advantages in the surgical treatment of some accidents and sudden illnesses, e. g., endovascular stent implantation for acute myocardial infarction, surgical treatment after traffic accidents. However, methodology of WM is mechanical reductionism, it ignores that life is an individual's overall characteristics, and is a very sophisticated system. Accordingly, WM focuses more on body parts than the whole body, more on the analysis than the integration, and more on physiology than spirit. In contrast, TCM is based on the Taoist theories of *Yin Yang* and *Five Phases* proposed in the ancient Chinese book "*Yi Jing*". "*Yellow Emperor's Classic of Medicine*" is the theoretical basis of TCM, and "*Treatise on Cold Damage and Miscellaneous Diseases* (Shang Han Lun)", "*Compendium of Materia Medica* (Ben Cao Gang Mu)", etc, are treatment techniques of TCM. TCM is a whole system involving theories and treatment techniques guided by the harmonic system theory between human and nature. As the old saying gose, human body is a small universe and universe is a big body, could give this implication. Therefore, the theoretical basis of life cognition in TCM and WM is entirely different, and there is no compatibility between them. Obviously, it is unfeasible to explain the curative effects of TCM by the theory and viewpoints of WM, and it is completely wrong to guide the development of TCM with WM theory. Therefore, the viewpoint of "Integration between TCM and WM" policy is worthy of debate and reconsideration.

In the field of medicine, in my opinion, TCM is orthodox medicine with or without the approval of WM. Many facts have proved that TCM can do a good job with skill and ease, and has achieved many magical curative effects in the cases while WM cannot. For example, hypertension is one of the common diseases of human beings. Hypertension is treated with various antihypertensive drugs by WM and patients always need to take medicine for life. However, from the perspective of TCM, the elevated blood pressure is the instinct of the repair function of body itself towards one local problem. A TCM doctor should find the location and cause of disease before treatment, and then have symptomatic treatment. I suffered from high blood pressure a year ago. If I took western medicine, I might need to take antihypertensive drugs for life. But one TCM doctor suggested me using crystal sugar, hawthorn and ebony to decoct in water and then to drink. Unexpectedly, half a month later, my blood pressure returned to normal, without any relapse so far. As another example, diabetes is also one of the common diseases in modern times. A man over 60 years old had 15 years of diabetes, suffering from the multiple treatments of WM. But the diabetes was getting worse, he even had serious complication. His venous thrombosis of the lower limbs made him almost lose the capacity to move. After more than a year of Chinese medicine treatment by Doctor Zhang, he has successfully recovered. The chronic kidney disease is also a common disease. when it come to renal failure the treatment by WM is usually kidney dialysis, and even kidney transplant, but the cure ratio is very low. In order to further prove the effectiveness and efficiency of TCM in the treatment of diseases, Dr. Zhang recruited 20 patients with chronic kidney diseases nationwide in 2016. Among which, one patient had renal atrophy diagnosis when Doctor Zhang diagnosed him, and Jianjun said that there was no chance of recovery and he had to give up TCM treatment. Another patient had no significant signs of improvement after one month of treatment. But the other 18 patients, got pure Chinese medicine treartment of threemonths after discontinuing all western drugs including hormones, and have returned to normal or maintained clinical maintenance standard for more than one year. Although the sample capacity is small, it is enough to prove the miraculous effect of TCM.

Doctor Jianjun Zhang is one of the few talent TCM doctors I have met. He was well educated in the orthodox surgery of WM in Nanjing Medical University, and had engaged in clinical surgery for more than ten years after graduation. However, in the face of the suffering of numerous patients and cognition of limitations of WM, he decided to give up WM and learn TCM. He believed that TCM would be the ultimate solution to human diseases. After many discussions with him, I summed here up his views on TCM: (1) Chinese medicine treatment of diseases is not only effective for chronic diseases with a slow cure effect as recognized by the general public now. On the contrary, the cure effect by TCM can be achieved immediately as long as the cognition of disease causes is accurate. (2) Chinese medicine treatment is based on the system theory, emphasizing the *Yin* and *Yang* balance of the body and the patency of the meridians. Therefore, a talent TCM doctor can cure all kinds of diseases rather than specialized only in certain diseases, because each disease is due to the body imbalance of *Yin and Yang* and the local meridian blockage. (3) For TCM treatment, if one pair of medicine contains more than 10 herbs, this prescription can be considered defective, and it generally does not require very expensive herbs. (4) *Yellow Emperor's Classic of Medicine* is the basis of TCM. We have deviated from the correct understanding of it due to the evolution of Chinese characters in the past more than two thousand years. Therefore, in order to correctly restore the connotation of dialogue between *Yellow Emperor* and *Qi Bo* (an ancient Sage in the field of medicine), we need to concentrate on the origin and the original meaning of each Chinese character. For this purpose, Doctor Zhang is still engaging in the study of the *Yellow Emperor's Classic of Medicine* and the original meanings of its Chinese characters.

This book Chinese cold—— *Roadmap to Traditional Chinese Medicine*, is the first academic work of Doctor Jianjun Zhang, which is more like a popular science work on TCM. In popular language, he clarifies the relationship between human health and universe motion, introduces in detail the basic theoretical models of TCM, that is, *Yin Yang* and the *Five Phases*, and four – Season – Six – Qi, as well as his own unique cognition of diseases and health preserving. In this book, Doctor Zhang used one Chinese herb – dried orange peel, as one example, to illustrate the efficacy of a Chinese medicinal herb is strongly related to its place of origin, growing conditions, climate and so on, and its suitability of the treatment for different diseases. The book is well written to introduce TCM with clear concepts, logical meticulosity and proper analogy. As a layman, I have benefited a lot from it. Although the book is a popular science work of TCM, it clearly shows the unique views of Doctor Zhang on TCM, e. g., he reasonably simplifies the human body into the two elementary units of energy (*Qi*) and information (*Ling*) , the same for the universe. These have obvious positive effects on improving our correct cognition of TCM. I sincerely hope and strongly believe that the publication of this book will greatly promote the development of TCM and help it to return to the right track.

Dean, Professor Dr. Gaowu Qin

School of Materials Science and Engineering,

Northeastern University, China

June 1st, 2017

秦

序

自　序

中医之理，源出周室，穷天人之际，究五行之变，载于《内经》，莫中华生命学之基。《内经》上终天气，下毕地纪，意在为后世子孙昭示阴阳变化之理，上以治民，下以治身，远离疾苦。

至汉代，仲景感伤寒之肆虐，伤横夭之莫救，悟《内经》之意，博采众方，作《伤寒杂病论》。从此立以草药治病之圭臬，仲景亦被后世医家尊为方术之祖，其功大矣。

今时之人，重有形之质，轻无形之变，重已病，轻未病，不知万事皆有前呈后启之理，致中医源流不显，万千疾病肆虐于世。身为医家，举目难见寿终正寝之人，百姓愁苦之状不下于建安年间。今不鄙浅陋，研读《内经》《伤寒》，写作《中医密码——医之源》一书，以求引玉，共承华夏医学之魂。

张健君

2017 年 6 月 1 日

Author's preface

The theory of traditional Chinese medicine (TCM), which originated from the Royal family of Zhou Dynasty two thousand years ago, makes a complete inquiry into the laws of the universe and change of Five Phases. The theory was recorded in detail in Yellow Emperor's Classic of Medicine, and has laid the foundation stone of Chinese life science. It provides the detailed informationfrom the sky to the earth, in an attempt to make clear to the Chinese descendants the change of Yin and Yang in the universe, with the intention of cultivating their minds, treating their diseases and keeping them away from sufferings.

Dating back to Han Dynasty when most people suffered from the cold damage diseases and died prematurely, Doctor Zhang Zhongjing who was unable to do anything about it mourned for the lost lives. Later on, after reading closely Yellow Emperor's Classic of Medicine and studied many prescriptions of Chinese medicine, finally wrote the medical masterpiece, Treatise on Cold Damage and Miscellaneous Diseases. Since then, the standards of treating diseases with herbal medicines had been set. And Doctor Zhang was thus honored by medical workers of later generations as the founder of TCM prescriptions due to his immeasurable contributions.

Modern people pay much attention to tangible matters rather than invisible Qi (energy), and do not understand that all the things present right now always had a long – term development process before and will indicate somethinginthefuture. Most people at present take the diseases seriously but ignore pre – diseases (sub – health). This tendency makes the superiority of TCM not well embodied and various diseases rage across the world. As a Doctor of TCM, I hardly see anyone with matured longevity, and most people suffer still from various diseases now, which is not better than what happened in Jian' an Period of latter Han Dynastywhen two – thirds of persons died of the typhoid fever. After carefully studying Yellow Emperor' s Classic of Medicine and Treatise on Cold Damage and Miscellaneous Diseases, I wrote this book in my own viewpoints, Roadmap to Traditional Chinese Medicine. This book introduces the truth and science behind the prescriptions of TCM, and I sincerely hope that it could trigger more comprehensive discussions and thus would save the essence of TCM.

Dr. Jianjun Zhang

June 1st, 2017

中医

密码——

医之源

目录 Contents

中医
密码——
医之源

无憾人生

A Life without any regrets

什么样的人生，是美好而无憾的人生？每个人的回答可能都不一样，因为这个问题是一个涉及生命观和价值观的问题，不同的社会文化背景会有不同的答案。在中国传统的观念里，达到五个标准，就是美好无憾的人生，这五个标准是："生命长寿、物质富足、健康安宁、积德行善、无憾离世"，俗称"五福"。中国有一个延续上千年的传统，就是在每年春节，每家每户门扇上要贴一张代表吉祥喜庆的红纸，上书四个大字"五福临门"，意在祈福，表达一家老小对世俗美好生活的向往。

"寿"为长久之意，为五福之首，所以把生命的时限，冠以"寿命"之称，隐含人们对生命长久的期望。与"寿"意义相反的汉字为"夭"，没有活到自然寿命而死亡，此为人生一大不幸。若用"长寿"这个标准考量人的生活，可以说我们现今大多数人的人生都不完美，因为都是一种因疾病而"早夭"的状态，寿终正寝的老人越来越少，基本上在七八十这个年龄段在医院的病床上离开人世。

根据地球上不同物种的生命周期特征，可以推测人的正常寿命应该在125－175岁之间，但实际情况是百岁以上的老人非常稀少，这就意味着大多数人没有活到天然年龄，此为"早夭"。这本是一件非常悲哀的事，但是因为大家把寿命的标尺定错了，误以为人过七十古来稀是正常的，所以没有觉察出"早夭"的悲哀。因此，人生最重要的一件事，如何长寿和如何保持健康，被大多数人忽视了。更有甚者，误以为养生保健是医生的事，在如何维持身体健康方面，过度的依赖医生，却没有发现医生的健康状况比之一般人，并没有显著的差异。

有人会说，80岁以后，身体衰退生活质量下降，不能为社会创造新的价值，生活失去了意义，所以年纪大了就应该离开。如果这种看法成立，那么不同的人对生命的意义有不同的认知，难道那些被认为没有意义的人生都可以被结束？80岁以后身体衰退的原因其实是不善养生的结果，而不是自然规律，所以追求长寿，如同欣赏冬天的美景，人生中每个阶段都有美好景致。

长寿有一个基础，就是身体的健康和心灵的美好安宁，没有这两个条件做支持，是不可能长寿的。所以追求长寿，并非贪生怕死，而是对美好生命的追求。长寿是美好的生活带来的自然结果，一个普遍短命的社会，一定是一个充满动荡暴虐和不安的社会。因此五福之一的"健康安宁"是完美人生的又一个标准。

在中国人眼里，物种的寿命，是上天设置的，所以尽享天年，是理所应当的事。不能因为大多数人夭折，就认为自己夭折属于正常的。就好像周围的人都得了抑郁症，而你没有得抑郁症，你反而怀疑自己是否正常一样。我曾经见过一个小姑娘，因为她周围的同龄人在月经前都会腹痛，而她自己却没有任何感觉，结果她找医生问，自己是不是不正常？

中国古人把长寿放在五福第一位，一是源自于对生命的尊重，快乐、财富、爱……都是围绕生命展开的，所以没有凌驾于生命之上的价值观，生存得更好本身就是意义，二是康宁、富足、好德、善终四种福德俱全之后，必然会产生"长寿"这个结果，所以"寿"居五福之首。东方的圣人在讲述《黄帝内经》里生命奥秘的时候，亦选择了以长寿作为切入点。

What kind of life is a happy life or a life without any regrets? Answers may vary from person to person because the question involves one's philosophy and values of life. People who have different social and cultural backgrounds will have different answers. In Chinese traditional concepts, to achieve five criteria is to own a life without any regrets, commonly known as *Five Fu*s(五福), a synonym for blessings, that is, longevity, wealth, wellbeing, benevolence and peaceful death. For thousands of years, the Chinese nation has carried on the tradition of praying for *Five Fu*s. At the Spring Festival, Chinese people paste up a piece of red paper on their doors, the red color symbolizing joy and happiness. On the red paper are four written Chinese characters(五福临门) bearing the meaning of the advent of *Five Fu*s, which convey the whole family's desire to live a wonderful life.

The Chinese character"寿(*shou*) "denotes permanence, coming top in the list of *Five Fu*s. So we call the life limit"lifetime", which implies people's expectations of a long – term life. In contrast, the antonym of"寿(*shou*) "is"夭(*yao*) " which refers to the phenomenon that one dies younger than his lifespan permits. It is a great misfortune befalling a person. Judging one's life by the criterion of longevity, it can be said that the life of the majority of people is far from perfect because they are usually confronted with the fate of dying younger due to diseases. There are fewer and fewer elderly people who peacefully die a natural death. Most people pass away in the hospital beds in their 70s or 80s .

According to the life cycle characteristics of different species on the earth, the normal lifespan of human beings is expected to be 125 – 175 years, but the truth is that the number of the people aged over 100 is very small, which implies that the majority fail to live up to their maximum lifespan. This phenomenon of dying younger(premature death) is actually a very mournful occurrence, but it goes unnoticed in that by the wrong criterion of life expectancy, it is taken normality that few people can break free from the bonds of human life expectancy of 70 years. The majority of people never give proper focus on how to keep fit and to live longer, even if it is of the greatest importance. Moreover, they take it for granted that health care is a major concern of doctors. Consequently, as for how to stay healthy, they depend too much on doctors and ignore that there is no striking difference in physical fitness between doctors and the ordinary people.

Some people may argue when a person reaches the age of 80, his body deteriorates and the quality of his life declines, and he can't make contributions to the society any more and his life becomes meaningless. Therefore, when a person ages, he should depart from this world. Since different people have different understandings of the values of life, if such a perspective is justified, should the so - called meaningless life be put to an end? The reason why the physical body of the eighty - year - olds deteriorates is not that it is caused by the law of nature, but they are not experts at keeping their body in good condition. The pursuit of a wonderful longevity is like enjoying the beautiful scenery of the winter and each stage of life has its own unique beauty.

Physical fitness and a peaceful soul are the prerequisites for longevity. Without them, one cannot extend his life beyond his normal span. So the pursuit of longevity is the pursuit of a good life rather than the fear of death. And a good life naturally leads to longevity. A society where people are generally short - lived must be one permeated with tyranny, turbulence and restlessness. Hence, wellbeing, one of the *Five Fus*, is another criterion for a perfect life.

In Chinese concept, the lifespans of species are predetermined by Nature, so living one's full span is natural and reasonable. One should not regard premature death simply as a normal fate for himself because that's the doomed destiny for most people, just as you harbor a doubt that you are abnormal when people around you all suffer from depression whereas you are spared by the disease. I once encountered a girl who came to me to seek medical help because her peers had a severe abdominal pain before menstruating but she didn't. She asked me with confusion whether she was a normal girl.

Ancient Chinese put longevity before the other four blessings for two reasons. First of all, it is out of respect for life. Happiness, fortune, love etc. are all centered around life, so there exists no value that can surpass life. And to live better, in itself, is the meaning of life. In the second place, if one performs with wellbeing, wealth, benevolence and peaceful death, then his longevity will naturally follow. It is thus understandable that the longevity ranks first. The Eastern Sages took the subject of longevity as a starting point when they revealed the secret of life contained in the classic, *Yellow Emperor's Medicine Classic*.

圣人之教

Enlightenment by the Sages

在中国古代，有一本成书于三千年之前的书籍，叫《黄帝内经》，它是一部专门研究人生命现象和生命奥秘的书籍。三千多年来，历代的医家、养生家、修炼家都在不断地解读研究它的内容，直至今天依然如此，由此产生了中国的养生修炼学，医学，针灸推拿，武学……这本书包含的思想和内容被尊为中国文化的源流之一。它记载的不少内容，至今为止，人们还无法完全理解相关的生命现象和生命规则，但是遵照它的理论和方法，却可以轻易地改善人的健康，延长人的寿命。

生活中大家会发现一个现象，人到了 50 岁以上，伴随着身体机能的衰退，会生出各种各样的慢性疾病，这些疾病成了寿命最大的威胁。人们对慢性疾病产生的原因做了大量的研究，不论是环境和食品的污染，还是快节奏的生活方式和生理心理压力，或者是遗传基因学说等等，任何一个原因或其总和，都难以圆满解释人普遍夭折的原因。

现代医学技术日益发达，其优势体现在紧急抢救和带病延缓生命。《黄帝内经》对人不能长寿的困惑以及疾病产生的原因是如何认识的呢？

在这部书的开头，传道者岐伯认为人不能尽享天年的原因，是因为人失去了对"道"的信仰和遵守，导致了疾病丛生和年过五十身体机能衰退的结果。中国几千年来有道文化的信仰，而《黄帝内经》是最早出现"道"概念的一部医书，这就意味着，懂得了道，才能获得生命的秘密，才能长寿，那么什么是"道"？

In ancient China, a book, completed 3000 years ago, is called *Yellow Emperor 's Classic of Medicine* (Huangdi Neijing) , and this book specialzes in life phenomena and secrets of human life. Since then, medical scholars, health preservation scholars and vital energy cultivator(Xiulianjia) through various dynasties were all studying and interpreting its contents, so do the people till today. Consequently the following Chinese subjects appear: health preservation and vital energy cultivation, medicine, acupuncture, naprapathy, martial arts and so on. The ideology and contents of this book are respected as one of the sources of Chinese culture. Quite a few contents, can yet not be understood completely till now about life phenomena and life rules, but if conforming to the theories and methods in this book, health of human can be easily improved and life span can thus be prolongated.

In our daily life, it may be found that with the deterioration of body functions after 50 years old, various chronic diseases occur and become a major threat to life span. Large numbers of studies have been made to explore the causes of the chronic diseases: environment pollution and food contamination, or fast – paced lifestyle and physical and mental pressure, or genetics and so on. However, any one of them or even all of them cannot successfully explain the cause of common premature death.

Modern medical technology is developing day by day, and its advantage is embodied in emergency rescue and life lengthening with diseases. While in *Yellow Emperor's Classic of Medicine* how to understand the failure of long life and causes of diseases?

At the beginning of this book, the preacher Qibo(an ancient famous medical scholar) thought the cause that human being could not enjoy full natural life span is that he lost belief in and conformity to Tao(the tenets for cultivating health) , thus leading to various diseases and deterioration of body functions just after 50 years old. The culture of belief in Tao lasts for thousands of years, while the concept of Tao initially appeared in the medical book *Yellow Emperor's Classic of Medicine*. This means that only understanding of Tao, can secret of life be achieved, and long life be enjoyed. so what is Tao?

何为道？

What is Tao?

在众多医书中，最早的"道"概念出自《黄帝内经》。

距今五千年到一万年之间，在中国中部终南山一带生活着一群种族，传说他们普遍长寿，多能尽终天年，我们称其为上古之人。他们能普遍享尽上天所赐的寿命，原因是掌握了宇宙的一个秘密，这个秘密被后世之人称为"道"。因为他们知"道"，而且行为处处与"道"相合，所以他们肉体和精神协调一致并且高度发达，形与神俱，故能长寿。

这种"道"在中国曾经作为普通的常识，代代相传数千年，衍生出了灿烂绚丽的中华文化，包括如何长寿和养生的技术。可惜的是，这种纯正的知识在流传过程中，在最近的三千年中，慢慢的被隐藏了起来，变成了少数人才能掌握的知识和技能。

在《黄帝内经》这本书里，岐伯说年过半百而衰的原因是后世之人失去了对"道"的了解，从而导致思想和行为上出现种种失误，这种错误的行为方式是违背生命运行规律的，比如贪图美味美色，暴饮暴食，透支体能，会导致健康和寿命受到损伤。岐伯告诉我们，上古之人长寿的原因是"其知道者，法于阴阳，和于术数，食饮有节，起居有常。"后世之人不能长寿的原因是"背道而驰"，这是唯一的原因。任何细节的失误追根溯源都是"失道"之后的表现。所以想健康长寿，首先要明了什么是"道"，以及阴阳、术数的知识，最后把这些知识落实到生活的方方面面，用来指导生活，如此便能得长寿之福。

何为道

在汉字里"道"的本意，是供人行走的路途，所以有道则顺畅通达，无道则蹇塞难行，由此逐渐延伸出了规律之意。意为掌握了事物发展变化的规律，按规律办事，就是与"道"相合，能达到目的，违背规律就是背"道"，背道则招致灾祸。

中国人对"道"的信仰，起源于5300年前的伏羲女娲时代。"道"来源于一张图，先天八卦图。"道"的内涵成熟于3000年前的西周时代，也是以一张图的出现为标志，这就是后天八卦图。在中国人的心中，没有什么权威是凌驾在"道理"之上的，所以中国人是一个有"道"信仰的民族。

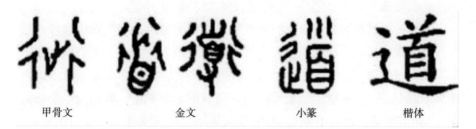

| 甲骨文 | 金文 | 小篆 | 楷体 |

图2-1　"道"的不同字体

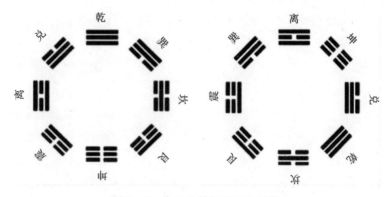

图2-2　先天八卦和后天八卦图

在中国人的传统观念里，人应当依据于大地的寒暑往来规律而生活劳作，繁衍生息；大地依据于上天的四气变化而有寒暑交替，化育万物；上天依据于大"道"而运行变化，排列时序，而与人的意志没有关系，它是自然存在的。归结为一句话就是"人法地，地法天，天法道，道法自然。"

在汉语言，使用最多的两个词，一个是"道"，另一个是"气"这两个字来源于中国人的宇宙观，一切生命都是道和气的衍生物，所以研究人的生命，就要要了解"道"和"气"的来源和意义，这是中国人研究生命的方式和视角。

中国古圣认为：有了"道"所以产生了阴阳之变，欲明白"阴阳"变化之理，就出现了研究"阴阳变化"学问的"术数之学"，有了术数之学作为理论基础，就可以研究人的生命规律，掌握了人的生命规律，就可以制定生活法则。

道是万事万物共同遵守的运动规律，所以"道"包罗万象，涵盖了万事万物。在中国人心目中，"道"无处不在，规律是凌驾于意识之上的，但不排除我们可以认识规律，并用自己创造的方式来描述它。这个描述的方法，就是东方"术数"，一个代表的概念就是"阴阳"。

万物因其道而生，所以我们要做的是认识生命规律和按照生命规律设计我们的生活方式。用从道中产生的规则来规范人的行为方式，就能保证健康长寿。所谓"德"，就是长期按照自然规律办事。知"道"积"德"。德积累的多了，生命就不会受到威胁，所以能健康长寿。归纳为一句话就是："知道全德，德全不危"。而术数就是用数理模型对"规律"的表达，就好像数学里的计算公式，所不同的是东方的计算公式用的是东方式语言。这就是天干地支五行八卦系统。这个语言系统的产生，来自于地球在宇宙空间的运行规律。

The earliest concept of Tao, among all medical works, came from *Yellow Emperor's Classic of Medicine*.

5000 to 10,000 years ago, in the region of Zhongnan Mountain, central part of China, lived some tribes, it is said that the people there generally had a long life and mostly could live full natural life span, and they are now called as People of Ancient Times. They generally enjoyed the full life span conferred by nature because they mastered a secret of the universe, and the secret was named as"Tao" by later generations. They were aware of Tao, and their behaviors conformed to Tao in all aspects, so their body and spirit coordinated very well and were well developed. Since their behaviors and spirits were all harmonious, they could live a natural and long life.

This Tao, ever as common knowledge in China, inheritance generation after generation for thousands of years, has created derivatively splendid Chinese culture, including the technology of long life and life cultivation. Unfortunately, this pure knowledge got hidden gradually in the process of inhertance in the last three thousand years and became a kind of knowledge and technology mastered only by a small number of people.

In the book *Yellow Emperor's Classic of Medicine*, Qibo(an ancient famous medical scholar) said that the cause of body deterioration over 50 years old was that people of later generations failed to understand"Tao", thus incurred kinds of errors both mentally and physically. These wrong behaviors were against the natural law of life, such as coveting delicious food and woman's beauty, and overeating and excessive consumption of physical energy, leading to impairs to health and life span. So Qibo told us that the cause of long life of the sages in ancient times was "they practiced Tao(the tenets for cultivating health), followed the rules of Yin and Yang and were in accordance with Shushu(the way to cultivate health). They had a balanced diet at regular hours, arose and slept at regular hours. "The only reason why people of later generations could not live a long life is to act in a wrong way even a opposite direction. Any small error is originally manifestation of missing Tao. So if one wants health and long life, first he should understand what "Tao" is, the knowledge of Yin and Yang, and Shushu (the way to cultivate health), and finally implements these knowledge at all aspects of the life to guide his daily life, so that the long life can be accomplished.

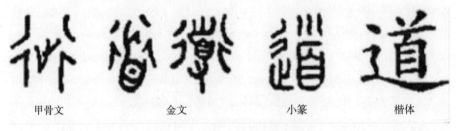

甲骨文　　　　金文　　　　小篆　　　　楷体

图 2-1　"道"的不同字体

What is Tao?

In Chinese characters the original meaning of "Tao" is the road for human to travel on, so it is unhindered and passable with Tao, while it is hindered and hard to pass without Tao . The meaning of Tao is extended gradually to the meaning of law, which means one masters the laws of nature under which things develop and change, acts in accordance with the laws, and he(she) should coincide with "Tao" and thus achieve the goal. Living against the law is being against "Tao", and thus will incur disasters.

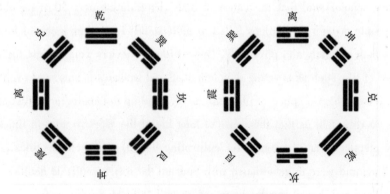

图 2-2　先天八卦和后天八卦图

The belief of Chinese people in "Tao" originates in the Era of FuHsi and Nüwa 5300 years ago. "Tao" stems from a diagram, Primitive Eight Trigram(eight combinations of three whole or broken lines, formerly used in divination) . The connotation of "Tao" matured in West Zhou Dynasty 3000 years ago with the appearance of a diagram, which is Posterior Eight Trigram. In Chinese mind, no any authority is above "Tao Li" (law, rule), so the Chinese is one nation with belief in "Tao".

According to traditional Chinese view, human should live, work, rest and procreate based on changes of four seasons on the earth. The earth has energy and information changes in conformity to changes of the four seasons to produce and nourish all things. The nature moves, changes and arranges time and order according to the great "Tao", which has nothing to do with human's will, and exists naturally. Summed up in one sentence, that is, "human must conform to the earth, the earth to the sky, the sky to the Tao, the Tao to the nature".

In Chinese language, the most two commonly used characters, one is "Tao", and the other is "Qi". The two characters originate from Chinese cosmology that all lives derive from "Tao" and "Qi". Therefore, to study of human life, it is necessary to understand the original meanings of "Tao" and "Qi". This is the way and perspective for the Chinese people to study life.

Chinese ancient sages held that "Tao" came into being, then there were changes of Yin and Yang. To understand the law of changes of "Yin and Yang" appeared the subject of Shushu. Since there was the subject of Shushu as theoretical basis, we can study the law of human life. Once the law of human life was mastered, rules of daily life could be made.

"Tao" is the law of motion commonly abided by all things, so "Tao" is all – inclusive and suitable for all things. In Chinese mind, "Tao" is ubiquitous, and law gose beyond consciousness. But we can perceive law and describe it with a creative way. This way of description is oriental "Shushu", and one representative concept for that is "Yin and Yang".

All things come into their existence according to their Tao, so what we should do is to cognize the law of life and to design our lifestyle conforming to the law. The rules derived from "Tao" is used to regulate the behaviors in our life so that health and long life can be ensured. "De" is to act according to natural law in a long term period. Practicing "Tao" will accumulate "De". When "De" accumulates sufficiently, life will not be threatened, so health and long life could be achieved. It is concluded in one sentence, that is, "Practicing Tao will accumulate De, more

De preserves health". Shushu is to express "law" in mathematical model, just like formula in mathematics, and the difference is that the language employed for oriental formula is oriental language, that is, the system of Tiangan Dizhi(Heavenly Stems and Earthy Branches) and Wuxing(the Five Phases) Bagua(the Eight Diagrams). This language system has been created in conformity with motion law of the earth in the universe.

天地合气，命之曰人

Species come into being by the
intercourse betweenQi of sky and
Qi on the earth

所谓"气"，含有能量的意思，能量长久有规律地交汇演变，就会以有形的方式表现出来，所以有形的物质其实都是能量的聚合体。中国古人说气聚而成形，形散而化气。万事万物皆是在一定时空条件下的能量的交汇聚集而形成的，所以世间没有一成不变的事物。人的生命也是如此，她的产生是天地气交而生，依据四时之法而成，故曰"生成"。此处的"人"，是人间万事万物之意，以人为代表来讲述一个道理。

以人为例，在个体生命的运行阶段，她也在不断地聚拢各种能量来维持生存。如果这个生命体处在一个良好的能量场之中，那么这个生命就是健康的。如果处在一个不良的能量场中，这个生命的正常运行就会遭受到负面能量的破坏，所以就会生病早衰。中国人称这个能量场为"气场"。一个人生命所处的气场，包括呼吸的空气，吃进的食物，精神情感环境，所有和生命有关的因素，所以建立良好的生态气场就是保持健康的手段。那么怎么判断气场的优劣呢，中国人有一套自己的运算模型，这就是中国的"太极"文化。

在中国传统的思想中，最受尊崇的人不是帝王将相，也不是英雄豪杰，而是懂得宇宙和万物运行规律，并能身体力行教化一方的圣贤之士。在中国人眼里，贤人通过学习，上懂日月星辰的运行规律，下懂四时阴阳物候变化规律，熟悉天地之气的变化规律，并根据历法安排生活起居，让自身的一切行为符合天地之道，并以生命的延长来体现自己内在的修养。

欲长寿，须知人的生命规律，欲知生命规律，须知生命的源头。如同江河之水，知道了源头才能知道她的流向和流域。中国古圣认为人以天地之"气"生，四时之"法"成，"气"为能量，"法"为规则。意思是来自于上天的能量，和地面的能量交互感应，而孕育出了生命，孕育出了最初的生命之后，这个初期的生命体随着天地之"气"生长收藏的周期变化，而产生出自己生长收藏的周期。人和天地遵从同一个规律，他们的表现形式不同，但是能量的运行规律却是一致的，就好像天地有一年四季，人有幼少壮暮四个时期，都是能量生长收藏四个阶段的表现。所以中国人认为，人体是一个小天地，天地是一个大人体，就是站在能量运动规律的角度上来说的。

那么，天地之气是如何产生的呢？

The "Qi" has the meaning of energy. Energy emerges and evolves regularly for a long period, and then will manifest itself in a certain form, so tangible matter is, in fact, an aggregation of energy. The ancient Chinese sages said that the aggregation of "Qi" would become a certain form of matter, on the contrary, the disappearance of one tangible matter would change into "Qi". All species are formed by emerging and aggregating of energy under certain conditions. So there is nothing immutable in the world, and so is human life. Human comes into being due to the intercourse between Qi of sky(Sky – Qi) and Qi on the earth(Earth – Qi), and grows up in accordance with the principle of the four seasons, so the process is called "Shengcheng" (birth and growth). Here "human" represent all species in the world, and is employed to state a truth .

Taking human as an example, in the evolution stage of an individual life, he is also gathering different kinds of energy to maintain his existence. If he is in a harmonious energy field, he is healthy. While if he is in a chaotic energy field, the normal existence of his life will be harmed by negative energy, so he will fall sick or ill and get premature senility. This energy field is called "Qichang"(Qi field) by Chinese people. The "Qichang" a person lives in includes breathing air, in – taking food, spiritual and emotion environment and other elements related to his life. Therefore, establishing good ecological "Qichang" is a means of preserving health. Then how to judge the merit of a "Qichang"? Chinese people have a set of operational models. That is Chinese "Tai Ji" (the Great Ultimate) .

In Chinese traditional ideology, the most worshipped persons are neither emperors, military and political leaders, nor outstanding figures, but the sages who know the evolution laws of the universe and all species, and who educate and civilize the general public. The sages are those who, by their own learning and study, know the evolution laws of the sun, the moon, stars in the universe, the change law of seasons, *Yin and Yang*, weather and climate. They are generally familiar with changing laws of Sky – Qi and Earth – Qi and thus arrange chedule time according to the calendar in order to make all behaviors fit for "Tao" of the sky and the earth and to embody their inner self – cultivation by extending their life spans.

To pursuit a long life, the law of human life has to be known. To know the law, the origin of human life has to be known. Just as water in rivers, only by

天地合气，命之曰人

knowing their sources, can their flow directions and drainage basins be clear. Ancient Chinese sages thought that human comes into being due to the intercourse of Sky – Qi and Earth – Qi, and grows up in accordance with the principle of the four seasons. Here "Qi" is the energy and "principle" is the law. It means that the energy from the sky and the earth has an intercourse and breeds the life. After that, the initial life produces its own period of *Sheng*(growth), *Zhang*(flourish), *Shou*(maturation), *Cang* (storage) with the periodical change of Sheng – Zhang – Shou – Cang of the sky and the earth. Human, *Tian* and *Di* all follow the same evolution law in different manifestations, but the evolution law of energy is consistent. Just as four seasons in a year on the earth, human also have four stages – infancy, youth, maturation and twilight years. They are all manifestations of the four stages of Sheng – Zhang – Shou – Cang of energy. Therefore, Chinese people hold that human body is a small universe, while the universe is like a big human body when it comes to the evolution law of energy.

Then how do Sky – Qi and Earth – Qi come into being?

天之道——日月星辰

The Tao of Heaven – the Sun, the Moon and the Stars

　　人站在地球上某个固定点抬头望天，会发现天上星辰的分布，在一年当中的不同时期是不一样的。我们把每次看到的星辰分布当作一幅星图，然后就会发现眼前的星图在头顶上一天天地慢慢移动变化，而且这种变化是连续性和周期性的。如果以某一颗星或某一组星辰为标志，就会发现它是从东边的地平线慢慢地升起来，又从西边的地平线落下去。过了不久，它又会从东边升起来，再次缓缓地下落。随着这一颗星或一组星辰的出现，同样的星图亦重复出现，就好像很多个星辰在一条固定的道路上行走，按时出现在一年中不同的时间段，这种天体的运动轨迹，我们把它叫做"天道"。那么天道对地球带来了什么影响？

　　中国人认为"道生万物"，道的本意是道路，因为道路是由很多人走出来的，可以直通目标，所以道又有了规律的意思。"天道"最初的意思，指的即是天体的运动轨迹。天体的运动是有规律的，就好像在一个固定的轨道上移动，随着天体的移动，地球上的万物也出现规律性的变化，所以把天体的规律性运动路线就叫做天道。天体在一条固定道路上周而复始的运动，反映的是地球围绕宇宙空间的某个点做周期性运动，所以才产生了星图周期性变动的规律。因此，通过观察天道，就可以知道地球上物质和能量变动的规律。掌握这个规律，对人类社会的生存和发展是非常重要的，否则人们连稼穑的时间都无法判断。

　　地球是一颗行星，表面是没有自生能量的，没有能量就不会在地面产生新的物质，更不要说生命。但是地球这颗行星围绕太阳旋转的时候，却在以年为单位规律性地接受来自太阳的能量辐射，所以地球表面就有了能量来源，就有了形成新生命的条件。

　　随着天体的运行，每当一些标志性的星辰出现在天空固定的位置时，地球上的四季变化就会规律性地出现。这样一来，星辰的变动就和地面上万物的周期变化对应起来，同时地上的万物也会在某个星图重复出现的时候，表现出特定的生长和活动状态。我们把大地万物的表现起名叫做"物候"，天空星辰的表现，我们称其为天象。物候的变动和天象的变动是对应的，所以掌握了天道运行规律的中国古人，抬头看天象就可以推知未来一段时间里地面物候的变化，从而安排农时和生活起居。

When watching the sky on a certain fixed point of the earth, we will find that the distribution of the stars in the sky varies in different period of a year. The distribution of stars we observed everytime is a stat chart, then we may find that the star chart is gradually moving and changing day by day, and this change is consecutive and periodical. After a certain period of time, the same star chart will appear again. When focusing on one star or a set of stars, you will find that they will ascend gradually from the horizon in the east, and descend to the horizon in the west. After a short time, they will ascend in the east, and gradually descend. Together with the appearance of this star or this set of stars, the same star chart will also repeat which seems like stars move on a fixed way and appear on time in different periods of a year. This motion orbit of celestial bodies is called "*Tian Tao*". What influence does *Tian Tao* have upon the Earth?

Chinese people think that "*Tao* produces all species". the original meaning of Tao is the road. The road is produced by walking of many people and can lead directly to the targets, so *Tao* has also the meaning of law. The original meaning of "Tian Tao" indicates motion orbit of celestial bodies. The motion of celestial bodies has regularity, just as it moves along a fixed orbit. Following the motion of celestial bodies, all species on the Earth are changing regularly. So the regular motion route of celestial bodies is called "Tian Tao". The periodic motion of celestial bodies along a fixed route indicates the motion of the Earth round a certain point in the universe space, and thus produces the law of periodic change of the star chart. Therefore, by observing "Tian Tao", we can know the changing law of matter and energy on the Earth. It is very important to master this law for survival and development of human society. Otherwise, it is impossible to judge the time for farming.

The Earth is a planet, and cannot produce energy on the surface. new matter can't be produced on the earth without energy, let alone life. But while the planet Earth travels round the sun, it receives energy radiated from the sun in a fixed period of one year. Accordingly, there is energy on the surface of the Earth. the conditions to form new life are satisfied then.

With the motion of celestial bodies, when some landmark stars appear at a certain position in the sky, the change of four seasons on the Earth will occur reg-

天
之
道
｜
日
月
星
辰

ularly. In this way, the change of the stars is corresponding to the periodic change of all species on the earth. Meanwhile, all species on the earth will manifest their specific growth and motion states when a certain star chart repeats. The manifestation of all species on the earth is called "*Wuhou*", and the manifestation of the stars in the sky is called "*Tianxiang*". Changes of "*Wuhou*" and "*Tianxiang*" correspond to each other. Therefore ancient people that mastered motion law of *Tian Tao* could infer the change of "*Wuhou*" on the earth in the following period of time by observing "*Tianxiang*" so as to arrange farming and schedule time.

阴阳之道——能量消长

The Tao of Yin and Yang – Growth and Decline of Energy

　　地球自转产生了以日为周期的昼夜交替，地球围绕太阳公转产生了以年为周期的寒暑交替，这是地球自转和公转引发的来自太阳对地球的能量周期性变化。中国古人为了认识能量之道，把地面吸收太阳能量的状态称之为"阳"，将能量辐射到地表空间的状态称之为"阴"，这样就产生了最早的"阴、阳"概念。

　　因为"阴阳"是描述能量进入和放出这两个过程的，而万事万物的产生和发展都离不开能量的输入和输出这个交替规律。所以，后来"阴阳"这个概念就作为思维工具，被广泛使用到对任何事的认识当中。"阴阳"概念来源于天体运动对地球能量的注入和地球吸收能量之后的散射，故中国的古人认为"道生阴阳"。有了阴阳就有了能量周期性变化，那么研究变化规律的学问。就叫做"术数"。术数之学虽来自于上古天文学，但是具体的运算却囊括了万事万物。掌握了这门技术的人就叫做"术士"，"士"在中国古代是对有学问者的尊称。

　　在中国各行各业里，曾经有过大量的术士，其中主管养生和治疗疾病的术士相当于今天的医生，他们用自己的术数之学为中华文明作出了重要贡献。

Rotation of the Earth produces alternation of day – time and night – time with one day as a period, and revolution of the Earth round the sun produces alternation offour seasons with one year as a period. This causes periodic change of energy radiated from the sun. In order to understand *Tao* of energy, ancient Chinese Sages called the phase *Yang* when the earth received the energy from the Sun, while they called the phase *Yin* when the energy on the earth radiated again to the terrestrial space. This is the earliest concept of *Yin* and *Yang*.

"Yin and Yang" describes the processes of entry and exit of energy, while germination and development of all species cannot go against the alternation law of input and output of energy, so later the concept "Yin and Yang" is widely used as cognitive tools in cognizance. The idea of "Yin and Yang" is originated from, due to motion of celestial bodies, the absorption of energy to the Earth and the radiation of energy from the Earth after that, so ancient Chinese sages thought "*Tao* produced *Yin* and *Yang*". Periodic change of energy is understood when the concept of "Yin and Yang" is established. And the study of the law of periodic change is called "Shushu(numerology or divination) ". The subject of "Shushu" came from astronomy in ancient times but the specific and detailed operation includes all things and phenomena. the persons who mastered this technology is called "Shu Shi(warlock) ", and "Shi" is a respectful title for the person who was erudite in ancient China.

There were a large number of "Shu Shi" in all walks of life, including those in charge of health cultivation and disease treatment, similar to doctors today, and they made significant contributions to Chinese culture. with their own science of "Shushu".

阴
阳
之
道
——
能
量
消
长

昼夜阴阳

Yang and Yin in Daytime and Nighttime

太阳辐射到地面的能量会随着地球自转而出现周期变化。面对太阳的一面接受太阳辐射即是白天，当这一面转到背对太阳光线时，就是黑夜。白天到来时，太阳从地平线上升起然后上升到最高点，地面接收到的能量由少到多积累，地面的温度逐渐升高，这是一个"阳"增长的阶段。到了下午地面吸收的能量以向外散射为主，这是一个"阴"增的阶段。因此昼夜交替实质上就是能量增长和释放的过程。

我们先以日为周期观察太阳对地球辐射能量的变化，最困扰古人的一个现象是：太阳早上从东方升起，傍晚从西方落下，可是当太阳再次出现的时候，并不是从落下去的地方升起来，而是从东方地平线在前一日几乎相同的地时间、地点再次升起。就好象一个人从前门口离开，再次出现时是从后门进来。从这个现象可以推断出，以地球为坐标点，太阳的运动路线是圆环形时，才会出现东升西落的现象。太阳的东升西落产生了昼夜交替，昼夜交替引起了阴阳变化。

现代天文知识告诉我们：地球自转的同时围绕太阳公转，在中国古人眼里，地球、太阳运动的轴心是北斗七星，坐标是二十八星宿，我们现在要了解的是昼夜阴阳规律，所以暂且把目光放在日、地关系上来观察。

我们生活在地球上，受地球表面能量变动的影响，所以地球上的阴阳规律才是我们关注的，故中国古人以地球为坐标原点研究天体运行轨道。这种为了认识方便而设定坐标原点的研究方式，是中国古天文学的一个特点，这种设定方法称为"盖天"论。和现代天文学的差别在于，中国古人把天象的变动与地球的能量变化以及万物行动规律放在了一个坐标系里，并不是以发现新的星体为目的，而是通过在这个天人合一的坐标系，把天体运行规律和地球万物变化联系了起来。所以中国古人对有学问的"士人"的要求是上知天文，下知地理，中知人事。

随着太阳的起落，地球表面的能量变化是一种什么状态呢？我们设想一下，如果太阳能量总是周期性的辐射到地球上，理论上只要有足够长的时间，地球温度可以不断升高，实际情况并非如此，而是维持在一个相对恒定的温度，这是为什么呢？

原来地球在接受太阳能量的同时，还在散发吸收到的能量，太阳刚刚出山，光线照耀到地球上，此时地面对太阳辐射的能量是接收状态，随着地面接受能量的增多，有一部分就会散发出去，既有"阳"入，又有"阴"出，吸收和散发之间有一个时间差。

上午以太阳能量的入占主导地位，下午以太阳能量的出占主导地位，从日出到正午是阳入大于阴出，所以地面温度逐渐升高，下午三点以后，"阴"出大于"阳"入，所以地面温度逐渐降低。能量的出入是相对平衡的，所以地球表面保持了相对平衡的温度。由此可知阴阳平衡是万物生存的又一个条件。

《黄帝内经》中阴阳的定义是：以地球为参考点，太阳的能量"所至为阳，所出为阴"。有了能量的吸收才有了能量的散出，所以"阴"和"阳"相互依存。阴阳之道是天地能量变化规律，天地孕育万物，所以万物自然遵从阴阳平衡原理，这是生命的基本原理，也是生活的基本原理。

人吃饭实现吸收能量和储存能量，然后通过日常活动，将吸收的能量释放出去，这是生理过程，包含的原理也是阴阳平衡。如果只有能量的吸收或能量的发散，或者是吸收和发散不能维持动态平衡，会导致人体阴阳失衡而出现健康问题。故维持人体的阴阳平衡是中医养生和治病的基本原则。

在《黄帝内经》里，古圣岐伯说"饮食有节，起居有常"是长寿的方法。其含义就是能量的摄入和使用要保持平衡，不可暴饮暴食；劳作和休息也要遵守规律。睡眠是积攒能量，劳作是付出能量，睡眠和劳作对人体来说，也是一种阴阳关系，所以起居要符合自然规律，以免造成阴阳失衡，缩短寿命。

The energy radiated from the sun to the earth is changing periodically with rotation of the earth. it is daytime for the side facing the sun and receiving the radiation of sunshine. In contrast, when it travels to the other side without sunshine radiation, it is nighttime. When daytime arrives, the sun will rise from the horizon to the highest point, and consequently the energy received by the earth will accumulate and the temperature on the earth's surface will increase gradually. This is the increase stage of"Yang". In the afternoon, the energy absorbed by the earth's surface will prevailingly release outwards. This is the increase stage of"Yin". Therefore, the alternation of daytime and nighttime is a process of increase and release of energy.

First we study the change of radiation energy from the sun to the earth with one whole day (including daytime and nighttime) as a period. The phenomenon puzzled ancients is that, in the morning the sun rises in the east and in the evening it descends in the west, but when appearing again it does not do from where it descends to the horizon but almost from the same place and at the same time in the east. Just as a person once disappears in the front door, but appears again from the opposite door. From this phenomenon it can be inferred that, taking the earth as the origin of a coordinate, the travelling route of the sun is round, so there is the phenomenon that the sun rises in the east and sets down in the west. And this movement of the sun products the day and night alternate, thus changes of yin and yang come into being.

modern astronomical knowledge tells us that the earth rotates on its axis while it revolves around the sun. In ancient Chinese eyes, the axis of the movement track include the sun and the earth is the Big Dipper, and the coordinates is the twenty – eight constellation. We want to figure out the law of day and night, together with yang and yin. So let's put our focus on the relationship between the earth and the sun temporarily.

We are living on the earth and bearing the influence of energy change on the earth's surface, and that's why we focus on the law of Yin and Yang. Therefore, ancient Chinese sages used to take the earth as origin of coordinates to study the traveling orbits of the celestial bodies. It's a characteristic of ancient Chinese astrohomy to set the origin of coordinates for coghition convenience. This study method was called"Gai Tian"theory. And its difference from modern astronomy is that ancient Chinese sages put change of celestial phenomena, energy change on the earth's surface and motion law of all species in one coordinate system. It's not aim to discover new celestial bodies but to connect, in one coordinate system containing sky and human, motion of celestial bodies with change of all species on the earth. Therefore, the erudite"Shiren"(Scholars) were required to know astronomy, geography and human affairs.

So as the sun rises and descends, what is the status of energy motion on the earth's surface? Let us suppose that the energy from the sun is always radiating on the earth periodically, so theoretically in a sufficiently long period the temperature on earth will be near that of the star. However, this is not the case but a relative constant temperature is maintained. Why?

The earth begins to absorb energy since the sun rises. As the energy accumulated, the earth will release some. That is, "Yang"enters while"Yin"exits.

In the morning entry of the energy from the sun is predominant while in the afternoon exit of the energy is predominant. From sunrise till noon, entry of "Yang"is more than exit of "Yin" so the temperature on the ground is increasing gradually. After 3:00 pm, exit of"Yin"is more than entry of"Yang", so the temperature on the ground is decreasing gradually. Entry and exit of energy are relatively balanced, and thus the relatively balanced temperature is maintained on the earth's surface. Thus it can be known that balance of "Yin" and "Yang" is an important condition for all species to live.

The definition of Yin and Yang in *Yellow Emperor's Classic of Medicine* is: taking the earth as a reference, the state where the energy from the sun reaches is "Yang"and where the energy leaves is"Yin". There will be absorbtion of energy and then there is release of energy, so "Yin" and "Yang" are interdependent. Tao of Yin and Yang is energy law of Tian and Di, and Tian and Di breed all species, so all species naturally follow the balancing principle of Yin and Yang. This is the basic principles of lives and daily life as well.

Human being absorbs energy and stores it by taking food, and then releases absorbed energy out of body through daily activities. This is a physiological process, and also includes the balance of Yin and Yang. If there is only absorption of energy or release of energy, or imbalance of absorption and release of energy, Yin and Yang will lost the balance and people may get sick. So maintenance of the balance of Yin and Yang of human body is a basic principle of health cultivation and disease treatment of Traditional Chinese Medicine.

In the book *Yellow Emperor's Classic of Medicine*, the ancient sage Qibo said it was the way for a long life to eat a balanced diet at regular times, arose and slept at regular hours. It tells that absorption and consumption of energy should be balanced and overeating should be rejected. And working and resting should also follow the natural law. Sleeping accumulates energy, and working consumes energy. The states of sleeping and working of human body are also Yin and Yang, So life style should conform to the law of nature in order to avoid imbalance of Yin and Yang and impair of life span.

阴阳之变与时间空间

Change of Yin and Yang And Time and Space

太阳位于天空中的不同位置，辐射到地面的能量强度是不一样的。为了掌握因太阳运动轨道变化而引发的能量变动规律，古人在地上立一土圭，以测量日影来研究。当太阳照射到土圭之上时，在阳光的对侧，就会留下一道影子。通过绘制出不同时间段影子的方向、长度，可以反映出太阳光照射地面的角度和辐射能量的强弱，也就间接反映了太阳和地球相对位置的变化，由此可以确定时间的变化。可见时间实质上是地球相对于天体发生空间位移所造成的能量改变，所以在中国古人的眼中，时空是一体的。

中国古人在"阴阳理论"的基础上创造了十二地支计量方法。十二地支既可以代表方位，也可以代表时间，它把时间和空间统一到了一个象术模型中。这种时空一体理论，来源于中国人从能量变化和天地运转规律来研究万物的视角。

更为神奇的是，在太极时空模型中，中国古人不仅把"十二地支"用在了计量能量消长之中，而且用十二地支划分出了不同脏腑经络在人体的空间分布区域，并发现了不同脏腑发挥功能的强弱时间点。这种把天地万物和人用同一个数理模型来认识的方法，逐渐发展成为中国医学非常实用有效的养生治病理论。但因为这套理论的失传，现代人对其的理解非常少，所以造成了多数人对中医的认识是既觉神奇又认为不可思议。

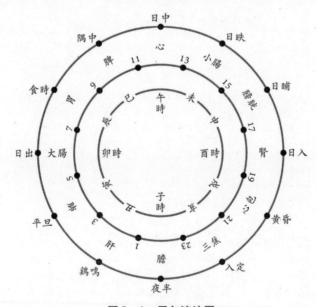

图 8-1　子午流注图

十二地支排序："子、丑、寅、卯、辰、巳、午、未、申、酉、戌、亥"。

十二地支中每一支相当于 24 小时计时法的两小时。24 小时是一个数字概念，但中国的十二地支计时法，同时包含了时间和空间，以此描绘了天地之间 12 种不同的能量和信息特性。我们到后面将会发现这种方式对认识万事万物起了执简御繁的作用，十二地支成了中国术数运算的一个基本语言。

Different positions of the sun in the sky have different radiation intensities to the earth. In order to master the energy changing law caused by motion along its orbit, ancient Chinese sages erected an earth sundial on the ground to measure the shadow. When the sun shines on the earth sundial, there would be a shadow on the opposite side of the sunshine. Then direction and length of the shadow in different time could be drawn down and reflect the angle and energy intensity of the sunshine on the earth. And the change of direction and length of the shadow reflect change of the relative position between the sun and the earth indirectly, which is used to determine change of the time. Time is, in fact, the energy change caused by the earth's spatial displacement relative to the celestial bodies, so time and space are a space – time continuum. .

The ancient Chinese sages created, based on "Theory of Yin and Yang", 12 Dizhi(the Twelve Earthly Branches) measurement method. The 12 Dizhi model could represent both position and time. It integrated time and space in one [*XiangShu* (image – numerology) model]. This theory of space – time continuum originates from a visual angle, from which Chinese people study all species from the energy change and in terms of motion law of universe.

More miraculously, in Tai Ji space – time model, ancient Chinese sages used "12 Dizhi(the Twelve Earthly Branches) "not only to measure fluctuation of energy but also to demarcate spatial distribution of various internal organs, and collaterals and channels in human body, and found the intense and weak timing when various internal organs function. This method of perceiving Tian, Di, all things and human with the same mathematical model has created a practical and effective method of health cultivation and disease treatment in Traditional Chinese medicine. This theory has failed to be handed down from past generations and modern people understand only a little of it, so most people deem traditional Chinese Medicine to be both mysterious and miraculous.

The order of 12 Dizhi is "Zi, Chou, Yin, Mao, Chen, Si, Wu, Wei, Shen, You, Xu, Hai".

Each branch of 12 *Dizhi* equals to two hours in 24 – hour chronometry. The concept of 24 hours is a numberical one but 12 – Dizhi chronometry includes time and space simultaneously, describing 12 different states of both energy and informa-

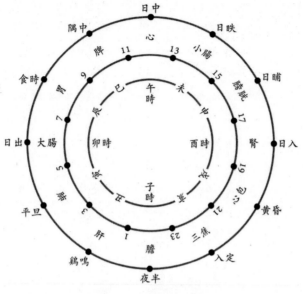

图 8 - 1　子午流注图

tion. In the following chapters we will find that this method plays a using – simplicity – to – serve – complexity role in understanding all species, and the concept of 12 *Dizhi* becomes a basic language in Chinese "Shushu" operation.

寒暑往来——年之阴阳

the change of seasons — cycle of Yin
and Yang take the year as an unit

地球在自转的同时，还在绕太阳公转，地球绕太阳公转的轨道叫做黄道。假如把地球设定为坐标原点，那么黄道也可以看作是太阳的运行轨"道"。因为地球接收到的外太空能量主要来自太阳，所以太阳是天道能量来源中最重要的部分，并以太阳运动作为天运的标识物，因此太阳相对于地球的运动周期，反映了地球最重要的能量周期——年。

这个周期是怎么形成的？它对地球和生命产生了什么样的作用？太阳周期和万物以及人的生命有什么样的关系？让我们一一来了解：

地球以年为周期绕太阳公转时，地球的赤道平面和绕太阳公转的黄道轨道平面有一个23°26′的"黄赤交角"，这个交角的存在，造成了一年当中地球在太阳公转轨道360°的不同位置。太阳光对地面的直射点是不一样的，用日晷测定发现，太阳的影子到了夏季某个固定的时间变为最短，从这一天之后，日影逐渐延长，到了冬天某个时刻日影变为最长，之后一天天缩短。影子最短的那一天我们称其为夏至，影子最长的那一天我们称其为冬至。影子长度的每一次回归，都代表地球绕太阳公转原点的回归，时间为一年。夏至和冬至就是太阳直射地球北回归线和南回归线的时间点。地球围绕太阳一周大约是360°，每天在轨道上前进1°，所以每天阳光对地面的直射点有或南或北的偏移。

每年6月22日前后直射点位于北回归线时，太阳对北半球辐射量最大，以此为中点前后的三个月就是北半球的夏季；每年12月23日前后太阳的直射点位于南回归线时，此时北半球得到的太阳辐射最少，所以天气寒冷，以此为中点的前后共三个月就是北半球的冬季。每年公历3月21日和9月23日前后，是太阳经过赤道的时间，在此之前的前后共三个月则是北半球的春季和秋季。这样一来，太阳对北半球地面的辐射从12月23日前后就由少逐渐增多。到了6月22日夏至，能量的辐射达到最高，从这一天之后，太阳直射点南移，北半球得到的太阳能量逐日减少，一直到12月23日前后（冬至）北半球接收到太阳的能量达到最低点。

纵观一年的能量变化，春夏以太阳能量的吸收为主，所以春夏为阳；秋冬以地面能量的发散为主，所以秋冬为阴。这就是以年为周期的阴阳变化规律。在中国人看来，人事的变化必须符合天地能量变化的规律，所以在养生方式上，他们有一个最基本的主张就是"日出而作，日落而息"，"春夏养阳，秋冬养阴"，以求达到人与天地同步的目的。

以能量出入的观点来划分阴阳，这是中国古人认识天地万物的一个基本原则，这个原则同样被用于与人生命健康有关的术数之中。阴阳理论如何使用？我们得从天地阴阳观过渡到生命阴阳观，才可以理解中医的阴阳观和阴阳理论。中国医家有句话，叫"善言天者，必验于人；善言人者，必本于天"，让我们继续谈天说地，丰富阴阳知识。

The earth revolves both round the sun and on its own axis. And the earth's orbital plane is ecliptic. When take the earth as reference, the ecliptic is also the sun's orbit around the earth. Because the energy absorbed by the earth is mainly from the sun. So the energy of the sun is the main source for earth, the sun is the most important component of energy source. And the"year"which is the most important energy cycle of the earth is associated with the cycle of the solar motion.

How this cyde formed? What effect does it have on the earth and life? What is the relationship between the solar period and all species and human life on the earth? Let me explain for you.

When the earth revolves around the sun, the angle which is 23°26′between the ecliptic plane and the equatorial plane is the obliquity of the ecliptic. The shadow of the sundial is the shortest at some day in the summer. It gradually become longer after that time. And when winter comes, the shadow of the sundial is the longest at some day, then it gradually become shorter. We called the moment when the shadow is shortest"summer solstice", and the"winter solstice"is the moment when the shadow is longest. It takes one year for the earth to complete the revolution around the sun. The summer solstice and the winter solstice are the time when the sunlight shines vertically on the Tropic of Cancer and the Tropic of Capricorn. One cycle of the earth moving around the sun is about 360 °in which about 1° for one day. so the subsolar point is moving towards south or north a little bit every day.

When the sunlight shines vertically on the Tropic of Cancer in June 22nd every year, the radiation of the sun is the strongest for the Northern Hemisphere. And the period of three months before and after the day is summer. when the sunlight shines vertically on the Tropic of Capricorn in December 23rd every year, the radiation of the sun is the weakest for the Northern Hemisphere, the period of three months before and after the day is winter. When the sunlight shines vertically on the equator in March 21st and September 23rd every year, the period of three months before and after the days are spring and autumn there. The amount of the solar radiation increases gradually since Dec 23. And it reach to the maximum value on June solstice. From then on, with the moving southward of the subsolar point. The amount of the solar radiation which reach the ground decreases gradually, and reach minimum on winter solstice.

Throughout the energy change of the whole year, the energy of sun is absorbed during Spring and Summer, called Yang, and the ground energy is be dissipated during autumn and winter, called Ying. This is the annually transformation between Yin and Yang. For Chinese people, human behavior should follow the rules of the nature. So they believe that "rising with the sun and going to sleep when it got dark" and "nourishing Yang in spring and summer, nourishing Yin in autumn and winter" are good ways to keep health.

To divide Yin and Yang From the view of energy in and out is one of the basic principles for ancient Chinese to understand the universe. This principle also applies to human health. If we want to understand the concept and theory of Yin – Yang in traditional Chinese medicine, it is very necessary to transit from Yin – Yang of heaven and earth, to Yin – Yang of life. Chinese physicians have words, "One who excels in Tao of nature must apply it to humanity to test it and adjust human health. One who excels in humanity must go back to Tao of nature to find the original principle and truth of humanity." Let us continue to talk and enrich knowledge of Yin and Yang.

寒暑往来——年之阴阳

天道左旋　地道右旋

The sun rotates clockwise while the
earth rotates anticlockwise

把地球作为一个研究对象，地球所处的外太空环境作为另一个研究对象，研究这两者之间的关系，就会发现，地球上向外辐射的能量，全部来自于外太空星体的辐射。太阳是距离地球最近的恒星体，所以太阳的辐射是地球最主要的能量来源。太阳对地球的影响有什么规律呢？

对于地球来说，来自太阳的能量辐射相当于给地球灌注能量，地球表面接受到的能量辐射积累到一定程度之后，再把吸收的能量发散出去。所以在天地之间，是有两股能量在此处交汇的，一个是从上而下的灌注，一个是从下而上的散发。从上而下的灌注就好像天呼出能量地吸收，从下而上的发散就好像地呼出能量而天吸收，这就是天地的呼吸运动。

地球由西向东自转的时候，相对地球上的观察者来说，就好像太阳的运行是从东向往西运动。站在太阳的角度看地球，地球的运动是从西往东旋转。当一个人站在天地的中间时，太阳运动的轨迹是从左往右，地球运动的轨迹是从右到左，所以天道左旋，地道右旋。

一个交汇周期里的四个阶段形成了地球四季，同时也规定了地球上的所有生命规律都由能量运行的四个阶段构成，而且天地能量的交汇创造出了生命DNA分子的碱基对和排列角度。所以阴阳螺旋式的交汇变化，能量的生长收藏周期是地球生命的共同法则。所以《道德经》有言："人法地，地法天，天法道，道法自然。"

黄赤交角，创造了螺旋形的能量交汇方式，螺旋形的能量交汇方式产生了能量的生长收藏，能量的生长收藏在水土的参与下，孕育了生命，这就是"一生二，二生三，三生万物"的意思。天道呼出的能量为一，地道呼出的能量为二，地道呼出能量携带了水分，所以天地气交之后生出了第三种能量。它不同于天能，也不同于地能，而是一种新的能量形式，并且内部有了生长收藏和湿气的参与，这就是五行的来源。

When we study the relationship between the earth and the outer space around it, we can find the energy that the earth exhales outwards is all from the stars in the outer space. The sun is the nearest star to the earth, so the energy of the sun is the main source of the earth. Then what's the influence of the sun on the earth?

As for the earth, the irradiation from the sun is like pouring energy into the earth. When the energy absorbed by the ground is accumulated to a certain extent, it will release outwards. Therefore, two kinds of energy interact in the terrestrial space, that is, one is pouring from the sun to the earth, which is like the sun exhaling while the earth inhaling. In contrast, the other one is exhaling outwards from the earth, which is just like the earth exhaling while the sky inhaling. That's the respiration of the earth and the sun.

For one observer on the earth, when the earth rotates from the west to the east, the sun rotates from the east to the west. But for one observing on the sun, the earth rotates from the west to the east. If a person stands between the earth and the sun, he might find the orbit of the sun is from the left to the right, while that of the earth is from the right to the left, so we say that the sun rotates clockwise while the earth rotates anticlockwise.

These four phases in one interaction period produce four seasons on the earth. This period regulates the energy change for all the living species on the earth, which also produces the base pairs of DNA and their arrangement angles. So the spiral interaction changes and the energy change period of flourish, growth, maturation and storage are the common law for all living species on the earth. As Tao Te Ching says, "Human conform to the earth, the earth to the sky, the sky to the Tao, and the Tao to the nature".

The obliquity of the ecliptic produces the spiral interaction of energy, and thus results in one energy change period of growth, flourish maturation and storage. Then it creates lives on the earth with the help of water and earth. That's the meaning of "One creates Two, Two creates Three, and three creates all species. ". The energy the sun exhales is One. The energy the earth exhales with water is Two. The third new kind of energy comes from the spiral intercourse between the two kinds of energy above, which is completely different from them, and has a characteristic of period of growth, flourish maturation and storage, and with the participation of water, *Five Phases Theory* emerges.

天道左旋

地道右旋

水土合德

*The earth and water run
harmoniously and regularly*

干燥的沙漠是难以储存能量的，太阳直射下沙漠温度会变得很高，而到了夜晚又会大幅度下降，这样的条件不利于生命存活。

地球上能出现生物，显出勃勃生机，一个重要原因是因为水的存在。占地球表面积百分之七十五的水域，创造了地球生命诞生的外环境。水是自然界大量存在的比热最大的物质，它吸收包括太阳在内的天体辐射能量并储存起来，又能把储存的能量以柔和缓慢的方式发散出去。所以在同一纬度，临海地区春夏温度上升的慢，秋冬气温下降的也慢。自古以来人类都是逐水而居，因为水能调节气候，滋生万物。

《黄帝内经》里说，地气升而为云，天气降而为雨，天地之间能量的交换是以水循环的方式来完成。《道德经》言"人效法天地而生"。水域面积占地球表面积的四分之三，水分亦占人体质量的四分之三，水循环既是地球生命的存在方式，亦是人体生命的存在方式。

《黄帝内经》用"发陈"、"蕃秀"、"容平"和"闭藏"四个词组为天地能量四个阶段的运行描绘了一张图画。

It's difficult for dry desert to store energy since it's temperature becomes quite high under sunlight and falls dramatically at night, it's hard to survive under such conditions.

Living species existed on the earth are full of vitality, one of important reasons is the presence of water. Seventy – five percent of the earth's surface is covered by water, which created the external environment of the birth of species on the earth. Water has the greatest specific heat capacity among the tangible matters on the earth, and it absorbs and stores the irradiation energy from celestial bodies including the sun, and releases the energy outwards in a slow and smooth way. So at the same latitude, the temperature at coastal areas in Spring and Summer rises more slowly than the interior regions, and falls slowly in Autumn and Winter, too. Since ancient times, human have settled down those places with adequate water, because water can regulate climate and breed all species.

As said in *Yellow Emperor's Classic of Medicine*, The earth – Qi arises to the sky to be clouds, while the sky – Qi sinks to the earth to be rain. And thus the rising and sinking of energy between the sky and the earth accomplishs by the water circulation. Therefore, as it was said in *Tao De Ching*, human was born by following the laws between the sky and the earth. The water area accounts for three quarters of the of the earth surface area and water content in a man is also about three quarters of the whole body. Therefore, Water circulation is the existing way not only for the earth life but also for human life.

The circulation of energy in the universe is described in *Yellow Emperor's Classic of Medicine* as four different periods with *"FaChen"*, *"FanXiu"*, *"RongPing"* and *"BiCang"*.

水
土
合
德

天地俱生——春

Wake up—spring.
Sky – Qi and Earth – Qi

每年冬天过后，随着太阳直射点从南向北回归。随着太阳逐日北移，太阳辐射到北半球的能量一天天增加。

太阳刚刚开始北移的时候，也就是能量开始"发"，地面还不会有明显的变化。随着天灌注能量越来越多，地面接受的能量由少到多，如同春天的泉水，从小到大，汩汩而出，能量开始在大地上分散开来，故用"陈"来描述大地接受能量时的状态。"发陈"形象地描述了天地能量逐日增长的一种状态，因为天地的能量同时在增加，所以这个阶段的能量特征是"天地俱生"。

此时能量还没有到达极点，虽然万物呈现出欣欣向荣的样子，但还没有达到枝叶繁茂的阶段，这是一个"阳生阴长"的阶段。《黄帝内经》中用"天地俱生，万物以荣"八个字描述了春天天地能量变动和物候变化的特征。

立春到立夏的三个月，从天空输入到地面的"阳"由少到多，把具有这种特征的能量形式起名叫"少阳"，主阳的生发状态。当这个状态维持到天灌注的能量到达极点时，地面能量积累到了最高点，地上物候的变化呈现出繁盛的状态，这就是夏季"天地气交"的能量状态。

中医
密码——
医之源

After winter every year, the subsolar point moves from south to north. As the sun moves towards the north day by day, the energy radiated from the sun to the northern hemisphere increases gradually.

At the very beginning of the sun moving to north, there is no obvious change on the ground because pouring energy is just to start("*Fa*"). With the energy of sky pouring more and more, the energy absorbed by the ground increases gradually, just like spring water turns out. Then the energy begins to spread over the earth, so it is used to describe the state of the earth's absorption of energy as "*Chen*". "*Fa Chen*"vividly describes a growing state of energy both in the sky and on the earth increasing day by day. The energy characteristic of this phase is thus called"Sky – Qi and Earth – Qi wake up(Tian Di Ju Sheng) ."because the energy at this period is increasing gradually.

At this moment, the energy has not yet reached the maximum. Although all species on the earth are nourished to born and grow up, they have not yet reached their lush foliage stages. This is a stage of"yin grows while yang is born". In the *Yellow Emperor's Classic of Medicine*, eight Chinese characters were used to describe the characteristics of energy change and phenology in the spring, "*Tian Di Ju Sheng, Wang Wu Yi Rong*", that is, the Sky – Qi and Earth – Qi wake up and all species on the earth are nourished to born and grow up.

During the lunar spring which lasts three months until the lunar summer, "Yang"poured from the sky to the earth increases, *Shao Yang* is called to describe this energy state, that is, the germinal state of Yang. As this state continues until the pouring energy reaches the maximum, the energy on the earth reached also the maximum. The phenology on the ground exhibits a prosperous state. This is the state of energy *Tian Di Qi Jiao* in summer, that is, the harmonious intercourse between the *Sky – Qi* and the *Earth – Qi*.

天地俱生—春三月

天地气交——夏

Harmonious intercourse between
sky – Qi and Earth –
Qi——Summer

立夏之后，太阳开始直射北半球，灌注到地面的能量开始达到高峰。同时地球因为积累了足够的能量，此时向外辐射的力度也增强。太阳的能量和地球的能量在近地空间的交汇呈现出一种旺盛的状态，《黄帝内经》称夏天的能量状态为"天地气交"。地球因为得到了能量的持续补充，所以此时地球上的万物处于一种能量交换活跃的状态。

就像一棵树木一样，春天能量来的时候开始生长，到了夏天能量积累到极点时，呈现出枝繁叶茂的景象，这个景象叫"藩"。内在的能量显现于外为"秀"，所以夏天是"藩秀"的状态，代表了天地能量旺盛交换。因为来到地面的阳从开始的"少"变成了最多，所以把夏三月能量积累到最高点，并且有旺盛交换特征的能量形式起名叫做"太阳"，"太"就是极点的意思。在水的参与下，食物链最底端的植物，在夏天与外界环境进行旺盛的能量交换，所以枝繁叶茂、生命力旺盛。人和动物到了夏天也同样进入了能量代谢最活跃的阶段。

《黄帝内经》把天地能量交换旺盛的夏季和地球万物在这种能量状态下的表现，归纳为八个字："天地气交，万物华实"。

Since the beginning of summer, the sunlight irradiates directly to the Northern Hemisphere, and the energy carried by the sunshine to the ground reaches the maximum in a year. The earth has thus accumulated enough energy, and gradually irradiates energy outwards at the same time. The interaction of the two kinds of energies derived from the irradiation of the sun and the earth becomes stronger in the terrestrial space. The energetic status in summer is called "Harmonious intercourse between the sky – Qi and the earth – Qi" in *Yellow Emperor's Classic of Medicine*. The earth has been continuously replenished by energy, so all the species on the earth is in a process of active energy exchange.

Just like a tree, when the energy of spring comes, it begins to grow. Up to the summer the energy accumulates to the maximum, the tree thrives with plenty of branches and leaves. This scene is "Fan". The inner energy is manifested itself outside as "Xiu". So summer is a state of "Fan Xiu", which represents the active exchange of energy between the sky and the earth. Since Yang on the earth increases from the little to maximum during summer, the energetic status of summer is thus called "Tai Yang" (greater Yang), referring to the energy accumulating to the maximum in the three months of summer and having active exchange of energy. "Tai" means greater or extreme. With the participation of water, the plants at the bottom of the food chain have an active energy exchange in summer, and thus have vigorous and luxuriant foliage. Humans and animals enter the most active period of energy metabolism during the summer, too.

In Yellow *Emperor's Classic of Medicine*, the active exchange of energy in summer and the manifestation of all species on the earth in this energy state are summed up as eight words "Tian Di Qi Jiao, Wan Wu Hua Shi" (Harmonious intercourse between Sky – Qi and Earth – Qi makes all species on the earth blossom and prepare for bearing fruit)

天地气交——夏

地气以明——秋

The earth Qi become clearer and stronger——Autumn

天空向地面灌注能量，假如没有一个界限，那么能量越来越多，地球迟早会变成一个火球。今天我们讲这些道理，因为大家有基础的天文学和南北回归线的知识，很容易理解。但是在古代，圣人向万民讲述天地之道的时候，只能用比喻的方法，而且是要用生活中容易理解的事件来做比喻。所以《黄帝内经》中，在第一篇里传达出万物运行规律皆来自"天道"这个思想后，又以"四季"物候变化的方式，来讲述"天地之道"和"天地气交，化生万物"的道理。

地球之所以没有变成一个火球，原因是这样的：

对于来自天空的能量输入来说，地球就好像是一个巨大的能量接收容器，从春到夏这个容器里的能量在一天天地变多，所以地上万物复苏并繁荣。但是太阳对地球能量的灌注不是无限增长的，上升到一个特定的值，就达到地球能量容积的极限水平。从这一点开始，天空不再输入能量，就好像一只无形的大手关闭了能量输注的阀门。

"急"在最古老的甲骨文中是用手抓住的意思，《黄帝内经》讲到秋天的时候，用"天气以急"描述天道下注的能量从这一刻起被突然收住，以地气向外发散代之。本来在暗处的地气此时发散到近地空间，由暗转明，所以此时天地能量的特点由"天地气交"变作了"天气以急，地气以明"。从这一天起，地球容器不再吸收新的能量。在一个短暂的转折之后，天地能量的交换呈现出地球能量向外发散的特征，就好像天空把以前输送给地球的能量逐日收回一样。

秋三月的天地能量特征，来源于立秋之后，太阳沿回归线南移，地面散发的能量大于天空输入的能量。所以总体上是地球储存的能量外出，天地能量旺盛交汇的夏天结束，转入到以地球发散能量为特征的秋天。

春夏我们以能量到达地球的视角来考察能量运行规律，关注的是能量的到来，所以以"阳"来命名春天和夏天的状态，阳从少到多为"少阳"，阳达到极点为"太阳"。到了秋季，天地能量总的趋势是以"出"为特征，因此以"阴"来命名秋冬的状态。立秋初期，地球容器里贮存的能量最多，地气发散的也多，所以我们把秋三月的能量特点称之为"太阴"。此时地面散发的能量最多，所以地表空间的温度还比较高。随着太阳直射点的南移，地气持续发散而没有补充，地面储存的能量越来越少，天气逐渐变得凉爽。到了冬季已经没有多少可出了，所以冬三月的能量特征为"少阴"。

Sky pours energy to the ground. If the energy increases with out limitation, the earth will be on fire. It's easy for us to understand today because the basic knowledge about astronomy and the Tropic of Cancer. However, in ancient times, Sages could only explain the Tao of nature by applying metaphors with daily events which were very easy to understand. Thus, in the first chapter of *Yellow Emperor's Classic of Medicine*, after expressing that the operation law of things comes from Tao of nature, the writer used the phenological changes of the four seasons to explain the"Tao of the universe"and"All species on the earth are born due to the harmonious intercourse between the sky – Qi and the earth – Qi".

The reasons why the earth has not turned into a fire ball are as below:

For the energy poured to the earth from the sky, the earth is like a giant energy container. As the energy in the container increases day by day from spring to summer, all the species on the earth experience revival to prosperity. But the energy will not increase without any limits. When the energy reaches a fixed value, namely the extreme of the earth energy capacity, the sky would not input energy any longer to the earth as if an invisible hand has shut down the valve.

"Ji(急)"in the ancient words inscribed on bones or tortoise shells in Shang Dynasty in ancient China means grasping something with hand. In *Yellow Emperor 's Classic of Medicine*, when talking about autumn, the phrase"Tian qi Yi Ji"(the sky – Qi has been grasped) is used to describe the sudden retreat of energy input to the earth. Conversely, the earth – Qi starts to dissipate outwards. As the original earth – Qi in dark places disperses into the terrestrial space, it becomes clearer and stronger. In this period, therefore, the feature of the energy between the sky and the earth changes from the harmonious intercourse to"Tian qi Yi Ji, Di qi Yi Ming"(the sky – Qi has been grasped and the earth – Qi has come out clearly and strongly). Ever since this day, the earth container will no longer receive any new energy. After a brief twist, the exchange of energy between the sky and the earth is characterized by the outward divergence of the earth energy as if the heaven takes back the energy that has been previously sent to the earth day by day.

The feature of energy of the sky and the earth in autumn appears since autumn begins. As the sun moves along the Tropic southwards, the energy dissipated from the earth is greater than the energy offered by the sky. Generally speaking, it

地
气
以
明
｜
秋

means that the energy stored by the earth goes out and the summer of the energy convergence of the sky and the earth ends. It turns into the autumn featured by the dissipation of the earth – Qi.

When we investigate the law of energy operation in spring and summer from the perspective of the energy that arrives at the earth, focusing on the energy arrival, we name the status of spring and summer "Yang". We call it "Shao Yang" as Yang increases(as in spring) and "Tai Yang" as Yang reaches its extreme(as in summer). In autumn, the general trend of the earth energy is characterized by "dissipation", thus we name the status of autumn and winter by "Yin". We call the feature of the energy of autumn as "Tai Yin". Because at the very beginning of autumn, the energy stored by the earth reaches its maximum and the energy dissipates outwards from the earth by a large amount, resulting in the quite high temperature of the near earth surface space. As the subsolar point moves southwards without any supplementation of Qi and the earth Qi continues to dissipate outwards, the energy stored by the earth surface continues to decrease. Thus, the weather gradually becomes cool. In winter, since there is very few energy left to dissipate, we call the feature of the three months of winter as "Shao Yin".

水冰地圻——冬三月

The earth is frozen with cracked ground——Winter

天地能量的交流，在地球大气层以内，是以水循环的方式完成的，所以水为生命之源。因为天地间能量的运动是周期性的，所以一年当中水循环也是周期性的。水循环现象的两个极点——汛期和枯水期分别对应于四季中的夏季和冬季。

雨的形成是地面水分蒸腾到天上，遇冷成云再降下的过程。雨量大小决定于蒸腾量的大小，水蒸腾的动力来自于太阳的辐射量，所以天地之间的水循环强度与季节有关。春天到来之后，地球吸收能量逐渐增多，所以雨量逐渐增大。春季如果是梅雨季，到了夏天就容易出现大暴雨，这正好是天地能量交换强度增大的一种反映。

到了秋天，来自太阳的能量逐渐减少，所以水的蒸腾量越来越少，气候逐渐变得干燥。立冬之后，地球储存的能量在秋天已经散发的所剩无几了，这时太阳还在赤道以南和南回归线之间行走，因而北半球获得的太阳能量减少到了极点，所以雨量也就减少到了最低点，到了一年中的枯水期。

《黄帝内经》有句话，叫"天气降而为雨，地气升而为云"，雨量的减少，意味着天地能量的交换在冬三月降到了极点，所以冬三月是能量输出的关闭和收藏状态，又称"闭藏"。地也不能给近地空间散发能量，因为没有能量的供给，大地的表现是万物萧条，草木衰败，气温降到了一年中最冷的时候，水冰地坼。因为没有从天而来的能量，地面的能量也散发得所剩无几，这时候的能量状态就叫做"少阴"。

对近地空间来说，水循环是大气层内能量循环的载体。天地运行产生的能量交替之变，在水的参与下，孕育出了万物生命。这些生命因天地能量而生，所以在他们自身的生命运动中，都遵守着能量出入和交汇形成的规律。这就是"阴阳平衡"和"四时阴阳"的规律。

一年分阴阳，阴阳细化有四时。根据能量的消长分别命名为："少阳、太阳、太阴、少阴"四个阶段，又叫"四时阴阳"。年有四时阴阳，日亦有四时阴阳。一日当中，平旦至日中为日之少阳，日中至黄昏为太阳，日落至鸡鸣为太阴，鸡鸣至平旦为少阴。年有春夏秋冬，日有昼夜旦夕，人有生长壮老，均是能量周期运动引起的四时周期之变。这是生命的基本特征。

"四时阴阳"是地球万物生命共有的能量运行规律，此能量运行规律表现为生命的"生长收藏"四个阶段。

The exchange of energy between the sky and the earth is achieved by water circulation within the earth atmosphere. Because the operation of energy between the sky and the earth is periodic, the characteristics of the water circulation are also periodic. The two extremes of the water circulation phenomenon – the flood season and the dry season correspond to the summer and winter in the four seasons.

The formation of rain is a process that moisture on the earth surface evaporates to the sky and cools down to form the cloud and then falls down. The amount of the rainfall depends on the evaporation. The driving force of water evaporation comes from the radiation of the sun. Thus, the intensity of water circulation between the sky and the earth is related to the seasons. After spring comes, the energy absorbed by the earth increases gradually, so to rainfall. If the plum rain period comes in spring, then summer is prone to heavy rain. This is the response to the increase of the intensity of the energy exchange between the sky and the earth.

In autumn, as the energy from the sun gradually decreases, water evaporation becomes less and the weather gradually becomes dry. After the beginning of Winter, as the energy stored by the earth runs down in autumn and the sun is still moving between the equator and the Tropic of Capricorn, and thus the solar energy in the northern hemisphere reduces to its minimum and the rainfall also decreases to its lowest point. The earth then comes into its dry season in a year.

There is a saying in *Yellow Emperor's Classic of Medicine* that "the sky – Qi falls to form the rain while the earth – Qi rises to form the clouds". The decrease of rainfall means that the exchange of energy between the sky and the earth reaches its lowest point in the three months of winter. Thus, the three months of winter means the shutdown and hiding status of energy output, named as "Bi Cang" (Shutdown and Hiding). At this stage, the earth can not dissipate energy to the terrestrial space. Without any energy supplementation, the landscape is a depressed image with declined vegetation, confronted with the coldest period of the year, water getting frozen and earth getting cracked. As there's no energy given from the sky and the earth energy keeps running down till almost none, the energy status at this period is called "Shaoyin".

水冰地坼——冬三月

For theterrestrial space, water circulation is the carrier of the energy operation within the atmosphere. With the participation of water, the exchange of energy between the sky and the earth gives birth to all species. As lives are born thanks to the energy of the universe, they obey the laws of energy input and output and energy intersection in their own life movement. This is the balance of Yin and Yang and the law of Yin and Yang in four seasons.

A year is divided into Yin and Yang which can be further divided into four phases. Based on energy increase and decrease, they are named as Shao Yang, Tai Yang, Tai Yin and Shao Yin, respectively. They are also called"Yin and Yang in the four seasons". A year has four seasons of Yin and Yang. Similarly, a day also has four phases of Yin and Yang. The period from daybreak to noon belongs to "Shao Yang". The period from noon to dusk belongs to"Tai Yang". The period from dusk to rooster crow belongs to"Tai Yin". The period from rooster crow to daybreak belongs to"Shao Yin". As one year has spring, summer, autumn and winter, one day has sunrise, noon, sunset, midnight and human has childhood, youthhood, adulthood and old age. These are all because of the periodic changes of the four phases caused by the periodic operation of energy.

"The fourphases of Yin and Yang"is the energy operation law shared by all life on earth. This law is manifested in four stages: growth, flourish maturation and storage.

生长收藏

Principles of growth, flourish maturation, and storage

能量"所入为阳，所出为阴"，天地之间能量的出入多少不同，造成了四季之变。春夏是进入的天气胜过散发出去的地气，好象天在呼出，地在吸入。为能量运行的少阳、太阳阶段；秋冬是地气散发出去的能量多于天气辐射进来的能量，好象地在呼出能量，而天在吸收。为能量运行的太阴、少阴阶段。

人多于出，"阳胜则热"，所以从春到夏天气逐渐变暖。出多于入，"阴胜则寒"，从秋到冬天气逐渐变寒。此为天地能量变化造成的寒热变化，符合中医人体寒热变化之理，同时是中医辨证理论的基本原则之一。

天地之气之所以能交汇是因为有水的参与。地气在上升的时候，带动了地面的水分，然后在地表空间与天气交汇，完成天地气交的过程。所以最初的天气是一道气，地球吸收之后发散出去的是另一道气。这道气因为是反射而出，所以携带了大地、山川、河流的信息，已经不同于最初自天而来的那道气，天地之气在近地空间螺旋相交，就生成了第三道气。这第三道气是天地之气交汇而成，其性质既不同于一，又不同于二，是新的气，而且有生长收藏之变。又因为有水的参与，周期变动的能量加之于水，就产生了新的物种。《道德经》里说"一生二，二生三，三生万物"即是这个意思这也就是《黄帝内经》里"人以天地之气生，四时之法成"的意思。

春夏秋冬的四时阴阳是以年为周期的天地能量交汇过程，且昏昼夜的四时阴阳是以日为周期的天地能量交汇过程。"阴阳"周期在人体，指的就是生命体内部能量运化的四个阶段：吸收、分解、代谢、排出。在一个阴阳周期里，生命内部吸收的能量从"少阳"阶段开始增长，到"太阳"阶段积累到最大；从"太阴"阶段开始大量释放能量，到"少阴"阶段能量的释放到达极点，然后再进入到下一个周期。这也是一个事物内部能量运动的规律。少阳、太阳、太阴、少阴之变引发了事物的生长收藏之变。

四时是万物发展变化的四个"阶段"，它来源于背后能量的消长运动。抬首望天，俯首察地，"春夏秋冬"四季之变是每个人都可以感受到的自然现象。如果古人要向一个人讲解万物共同规律，以及背后隐藏的能量之变，采用春夏秋冬物候变化来举例说明，不是最好的选择吗？这就是古人的智慧。

年有四时——春夏秋冬，日有四时——昼夜昏晓，人有四时——生长壮老，万物有四时——生长收藏。

"少阳"、"太阳"、"太阴"、"少阴"四气分别对应于"生"、"长"、"收"、"藏"四个阶段。中国古人又借用四种物质形态来对应于四种能量状态，这四种物质形态是"木"、"火"、"金"、"水"。少阳为木，太阳为火，太阴为金，少阴为水，生长收藏构成一个周期。这个周期作用的原点是大地，大地为土，有了周期能量的参与，加上湿土，就变成了木火土金水五种物质形态。湿土有化育之功，此为中医"五行"学说的来历。

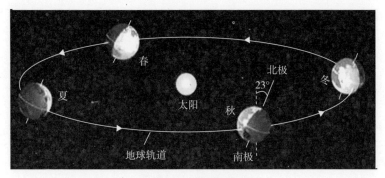

图 16 - 1　四季变化图

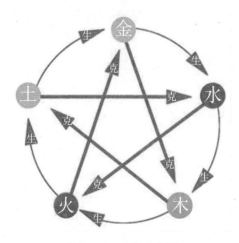

图 16 - 2　五行生克图

中医术数体系里，用"木火土金水"五行，来分别指代具备少阳之气的生态，具备太阳之气的旺态，具备运化之气的土态，具备太阴之气的收态和具备少阴之气的藏态。这样做的好处是把具有同等属性的万事万物，从能量运行的角度加以归类划分。比如春天具有木的属性，人生的少年时代，朝阳初升的早晨，以及一切事物的初起阶段，在五行属性上有同样的特性。这样可以抛开现象看到事物的能量属性，从而知道它的发展方向以及和其他四行之间的关系。

在中国古老的术数体系里，"阴阳五行"是描述万物规律的专有名词，任何事物从能量的角度都可以划归到五行中的一类。所以古人说，万物都在天地之内，五行之中。

Taking the earth as a reference, we can regard the state that energy coming to the earth from the sky as *Yang*, and regard the energy leaving away from the earth as *Yin*. The difference in the quantity of energy coming into and leaving outwards results in the change of four seasons. In spring and summer, the incoming energy from sky (*sky − Qi*) is quantitatively more than that emanating from the earth (*earth − Qi*). Spring and summer are thus regarded as the *Shao − yang* and *Tai − yang* stages of energy transformation, respectively. In contrast, as for autumn and winter, the amount of energy emanating from the earth is more than that incoming from the sky. Autumn and winter are thus regarded as *Tai − yin* and *Shao − yin* stages of energy transformation, respectively.

When the incoming energy is more than the energy emanating outwards, we call this state as *Yang* over *Yin* and it will lead to the accumulation of heat. Therefore, it gradually warms from spring to summer. When the incoming energy is less than the energy emanating, this state is called *Yin* over *Yang*, it will lead to the dissipation of heat. Thus it gradually becomes cold from autumn to winter. This is the change between the cold and the hot state arising from the energy fluctuation between the earth and the sky, in accordance with the change of the cold and the hot state in human body in Traditional Chinese Medicine. This is one of the basic principles in the diagnosis of TCM.

The harmonious intercourse between sky − Qi and earth − Qi is due to the participation of water. When the earth − Qi rises upwards together with the water of ground, it converges with the sky − Qi in the terrestrial space and thus completes their harmonious intercourse. Therefore, the first Qi is the initial sky − Qi which is one kind of Qi mainly from the sun, and the Qi absorbed by the earth and then emanating outwards is the second one. The later Qi contains the sufficient information of land, mountains, rivers and seas because it is reflected, and is completely different from the initial sky − Qi. The third Qi is born due to spiral intersection between the sky − Qi and the earth − Qi in the terrestrial space. The third Qi is a new one and generated by the intercourse between the sky − Qi and the earth − Qi. And it embodies the change of growth, flourish maturation and storage. It is different from both the sky − Qi and the earth − Qi. And because of the participation of water, the energy fluctuation in a regular period acts on water,

生
长
收
藏

and thus leads to birth of new species. Just like what *Tao Te Ching* said: "One creates two, two create three, three create all species on the earth", and it is exactly the same meaning described in *Yellow Emperor's Classic of Medicine*, human would come into being due to the intercourse between *Sky − Qi* and *Earth − Qi*, and grow up in accordance with the principle of the four seasons.

The four seasons of spring, summer, autumn and winter are the results of intercourse of *Yin* and *Yang* energy between the sky and the earth in a period of one year, and the four stages of sunrise, noon, sunset and midnight are the results of intercourse of *Yin* and *Yang* energy between the sky and the earth in a period of one day. Similarly, the periodical Yin and Yang in body refer to the internal energy period of absorption, decomposition, metabolism and excretion. In one period of Yin and Yang, the energy absorbed by body begins to grow up during Shao − yang stage until reaches the maximum, Tai − yang state. Vast energy begins to dissipate at Tai − yin state, and the release of energy reached the maximum in Shao − yin stage. Then, the next period repeats just like the yin and yang run in a cycle. This is also a universal rule of energy motion inside a body. The change of Shao − yang, Tai − yang, Tai − yin and Shao − yin induces the periodical change of growth, flourish maturation and storage of species.

The four periods represent the four stages of the evolution of all species. The evolution is due to a common mechanism of the accumnlation and dissipation of energy. Observing the sky and earth, we can find that the change of four seasons is a natural phenomenon which everybody can feel. If ancient sages wanted to tell one person the universal rules of all things and the change of energy hidden behind, wouldn't it be the best choice to take the change of seasonal phenology as examples? This is our ancient sages' intelligence.

A year has four periods—spring, summer, autumn and winter. A day has four periods—sunrise, noon, sunset and midnight. Human life have four periods—child, youth, adult and old age. All species have four periods, growth, flourish maturation and storage.

Four states of Qi, named Shao − yang, Tai − yang, Tai − yin and Shao − yin correspond to the four periods of growth, flourish maturation and storage. Chinese ancient sages also used four states of matters, Wood, Fire, Metal and Water, to de-

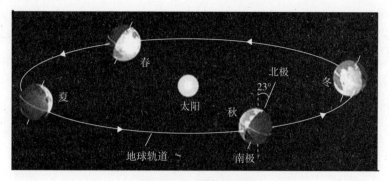

图 16-1　四季变化图

scribe the four energy states. Thus Wood represents Shao – yang, Fire represents Tai – yang, Metal represents Tai – yin and Water represents Shao – yin. And thus each state of growth, flourish maturation and storage consist of a single period. The original point is the ground, which represented by earth. With the participation of periodical energy and with the help of water and Earth, it is thus composed of five phases of matters of Wood, Fire, Soil, Metal and Water.

生长收藏

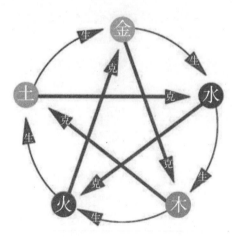

图 16-2　五行生克图

In the mathematical system of traditional Chinese medicine, the five phases (*Wood, Fire, Earth, Metal* and *Water*) represent the growth state of *Shao – yang Qi*, the flourishing state of *Tai – yang Qi*, the transformation and nourishing states of the earth, the declining state of *Tai – yin Qi*, and the domancy state of *Shao – yin Qi*, respectively. The advantage of this methodology is to classify everything of the universe with the same energy state into one category. Taken the *Wood* phase as one example, spring has the *Wood* characteristic, which is the same as the teen-age, the sunrise in the morning and the initial stage of everything. In a word, they all have the same characteristic—the growth characteristic of *Wood* by the *Five – Phase* theory. In such way, we can cast aside the phenomena and catch their nature of energy, and thus know their evolution directions and the relationship with the other four phases.

In the ancient Chinese mathematical system, "*Yin Yang* and *Five Phases*" are special and proper concepts to describe the universal laws. Everything in this world can be classified into one phase from the viewpoint of energy. Therefore, the ancient sages said that everything in the universe was controlled by laws revealed in the *Five – phase* theory.

善言天者必验于人（一）
——四时阴阳与人体健康

Tao of nature applies also to human beings——Yin -yang of the four seasons and human health

生长收藏是一个完整的周期，每个阶段都必须完成其或藏或发，或生或收的使命，才能形成一个正常和谐的生命周期。任何一个阶段的欠缺，都会影响到周期的完整。假如春天气候异常，气温该暖却寒，俗称倒春寒，那么到了秋季则果木难成。这说明能量运行周期里，一个阶段没有完成，则整个周期循环都将受到影响。

1. 四时阴阳与睡眠障碍

很多人羡慕孩子那种香甜的睡眠，而不少成年人会有睡眠不深的困扰。导致睡眠质量下降的诱因各种各样，以四时阴阳的观点来看，睡眠不深如同冬天的收藏没有降到最低点，就好像日周期中太阳该落山却没有落山一样，这是人体阴阳周期失常的反映。夜晚没有收藏，到了生发的阶段，生长之力就会不足。长此以往，人体四时阴阳不调就会导致健康受损。所以对人体来说，代表冬天收藏的充足良好的睡眠，和代表夏天释放的积极旺盛的活动，是健康的两个必要条件。古人以"动生静养"四个字，概括了保持人体四时阴阳周期的和谐之法。

长期熬夜的人因为收藏不足，所以精力会逐渐变差，改善的方法就是按时休息停止熬夜。同理，缺少运动或无所事事者，也会出现睡眠不佳的情况，这是因为白天没有生发到最高点，到了夜里就收藏不到最低点。针对这种睡眠障碍，有一个方法就是让患者在白天做一些高强度的体力活动。通过体力活动，让身体内外能量的交流达到最高点，完成"太阳"阶段的发散功能。到了夜里，睡眠自然就会变得深沉。这种现象和对治方法，来源于身体四时循环之理。

同理，只有夜里休息得足够好，第二天才会精神饱满。太阳之气对应于四季中的夏天，夏天的特征是火和热。少阴之气对应于四季中的冬天，冬天的特征是水和冰。人体的水火分别以"肾水"和"心火"代之。这里的"心火"和"肾水"非解剖学上有形的心脏和肾脏，而是虚指一种能量生长收藏的功能。人体四时周期的理想状态被称作"水火既济，心肾相交"。为什么能量的周期运动被称为"心肾相交"？在五藏与五行篇我们将讲述中医四时阴阳与五行以及人体结构功能之间的关系。

2. 一生四时

少年

因为四时阴阳是地球万物共有的规律，所以四时阴阳的术数模型可以用于研究任何事物。对应人的一生，四时阴阳可以分为少年、青年、壮年和老年四个阶段，对应于能量周期的少阳、太阳、太阴和少阴阶段。

少儿阶段相当于人生的春天，万物始发，天性柔弱。这个时候是积累能量的生长阶段，随着天地之间能量一天天的积累，草木吸收和感应了天地的能量与信息，开始慢慢地发生变化。经过发芽、开花和抽穗，草木由柔弱变得苗壮。草木在春天主生长而不结果实，经过夏的繁茂，到了秋的收降，植物内部的能量积累到达了极限，在本身所带基因信息的作用下，储存的能量转化为成熟的果实，为下一个生命周期做好准备。

处在发育期的少儿如同春天刚刚发芽的草木般柔弱，所以在生理和心理上需要有充足的保护。《黄帝内经》从四时能量的运行规律推导出一句话，即当一个人处在少阳阶段的时候，养育的原则是"生而勿杀，予而勿夺"。

少儿的养育方式，要多采用鼓励和引导的手段，令其生发，鼓励他们探索未知。在安全范围内，不要做过多的限制，否则会扼杀孩子的天性。倘若孩子行为有失误，也要善加引导，让他们在温和善意的氛围中积蓄能量修正成长，顺利过渡到枝繁叶茂的青年时代。对孩子的教育既不可采用过激的惩罚手段，也不可令孩子在肉体和精神上承载过重的负担。

孩子的天性与少阳特性相符，所以在生活中我们会发现孩子是最喜欢表扬鼓励的，越表扬他表现得越好。反之严厉的批评限制，或是采用威胁压制这样的杀伐手段，让孩子遵从大人的意志，会斫杀孩子的少阳之气，可能导致生理和心理疾病。

因为孩子未进入成年社会，所以对待孩子，不能与对待成年人一样，尤其是不能以成年人的价值观去判断孩子的好坏。只要能健康成长，不给他人制造麻烦，就是好孩子。很多伟大的人物在他们年少时候，都曾被当做弱智儿童。如果有人要求一棵树苗在春天结出果实，错在此人而不在树苗。很多家长望子成龙，希望孩子的一切都要符合大人的要求并且达到优秀级别。学习成绩要好，待人要彬彬有礼，甚至行住坐卧一切都要符合规范。这种按照成年人规范和价值观对孩子的期待、要求，可能会严重伤害到孩子的身心健康。

如果伤了春天的少阳之气，到了青年就不能正常转入到活力四射、积极上进的太阳阶段。能量的周期运行，一个阶段没有完成，就会影响到下一个阶段。就好像火车延误，这一站没赶上，那么下一站也不能准时到达，依次类推，这趟列车可能就没法预计它未来的行程了。

青年

青年时期，相当于一年中的夏季，此时地面接受的能量到达一个极点。天地气交旺盛，草木枝繁叶茂，身体内的细胞同时呈现出旺盛的代谢状态，人与外界的能量和信息交流达到了一个极点。所以青年时代是体能、精神、情感和智力发展的巅峰状态，同时也是情感最丰富、最适合谈情说爱的时期，因为恋爱是最强烈的信息交换方式之一。所以青年时代的恋爱，通常是最深的回忆。

夏天和青年时代是大量吸收外部能量，又大量发散储存于内部能量的阶段。所以青年时期，人的行为也要顺应人生之夏这个特征，大量接收外界信息，通过思想的碰撞交流来丰富自身。这个阶段的生活和行为方式是一种以交流碰撞为主的模式，所以大学阶段才是学习能力最旺盛的阶段，而不是幼儿园和小学。

青年人喜欢参加各种社会活动而不喜欢和曾经照顾约束自己的长辈待在一起，这是太阳阶段的能量特性所致。所以妈妈们不要因为孩子有了自己的生活而有失落感，这说明你的孩子开始进入人生的夏天了。假如这个阶段他还如幼年一样依赖于你，那才是麻烦呢。

中国古代养生家在谈到夏天养生原理的时候，打了一个有趣的比方，就好比你喜欢的东西留在了户外，总想出去而不愿意宅在房子里，这是体内的能量要发散不要收藏的外在反映。聚会、交友、社团、远行、恋爱等都是青年人喜欢的社交方式。如果人为地抑制了这个过程，那么就可能会出现生理和心理方面的问题。精神疾患的发病率在青年人中最高，与这个时期的社交以及恋爱受阻有关。所以对待年轻人的恋爱，最忌讳棒打鸳鸯。

没有春天充分的吸收，就没有夏天旺盛的交换。青年时代缺少与外界沟通的欲望和动力，源于少年时代春天少阳之气的不足。现在中国社会出现的宅男宅女现象，源于儿童和少年时代学校教育体制和家长不当的教育方式对孩子少阳之气的遏制。

没有夏天旺盛的交换，就没有秋天枝头的累累硕果，四时阴阳中如果一个阶段的任务都没有完成，到了收藏的阶段，人生难免会有遗憾。带有遗憾的老年，在中国人眼里，就是不能"善终"之意。所以人生的不同阶段，各自有要完成的任务，春华秋实，每个阶段都应该遵从四时能量运行的规律。

The period of growth, flourish maturation and storage is a complete cycle. Every phase has to complete its own mission of growth or maturation, flourish or storage, and thus a normal harmonious lifecycle can be formed. Defection of any phase will affect the integrity of the cycle. If the climatic anomaly occurs in spring, which is commonly known as cold spell in later spring when it's getting cold in an otherwise spring, the harvest may be hurt in the fall. This suggests if the task in one phase is not fulfilled, then the entire cycle will be affected.

1. *Yin – yang* of the four seasons and sleep disorders

Many people envy children who have sound sleep and quite a few adults are troubled by poor sleep. Various factors lead to the decline in sleep quality. From the perspective of *Yin* and *Yang*, poor sleep is a reflection of the abnormal period of *Yin* and *Yang* in the human body. Just as the dormancy in winter does not drop to its lowest point or the sun does not set when it's time to set, all these phenomena have something to do with the balance of yin and yang. Without good sleep (means good state of storage) at night, when it reaches the phase of energy dispersing, the power will be inadequate. In the long run, the imbalance of *Yin* and *Yang* in the human body will impair health. Therefore, for the body, sleeping time is embodied similarly in winter while energetic daytime is comparable to summer, which are two prerequisites for good health. Ancient Chinese generalized the way to keep *Yin* and *Yang* in *move to be active while meditation to rejuvenate*.

Those who stay up late in a long time basis gradually become less energetic because of the deficiency. The way to improve it is to go to bed early and stop staying up late. Likewise, those who lack exercises or idle about all day long are likely to have poor sleep at night. This is because *Tai – yang* does not rise to the highest point in the daytime and fails to drop to the lowest point at night. To solve this kind of sleep disorder, one way is to make the patients do some physical activities of high intensity in the day. Through physical activities, the exchange of energies inside and outside the body reaches its peak to bring the function of *Tai – yang* to its full play. At night, sleep naturally becomes deep. The symptom and its cure stem from the principle of the periodical circulation of bodily *Yin* and *Yang* in the four seasons.

Likewise, only if one sleeps well enough at night, can he or she be energetic the next day. Qi of *Tai – yang* corresponds to the summer of the four seasons, which is characterized by fire and heat, and *Qi* of *Shao – yin* corresponds to the winter with the characteristics of water and freezing cold. Water and fire of the human body are replaced respectively by"kidney water"and"heart fire", which have nothing to do with the tangible organs of heart or kidney in anatomical terms, but refer to the functions of energy: growth, flourish maturation and storage. The ideal state of the four seasonal periods of the human body is referred to a condition in which"the harmony between water and fire is achieved by the intercourse between heart and kidney". Why is the periodic operation of energy called"the intercourse between heart and kidney"? In the chapter of *Five Zang – viscera and Five Phases*, the relationships of *Si – shi yin – yang* and *five phases* of TCM, and the structure and function of human body are elaborated.

2. Four stages of life

Childhood

Yin and *yang* of four seasons is the common law that all species on the earth comply with, so its *Shushu* mode can be applied to researching everything. As for man's lifetime *yin* and *yang* of four seasons can be divided into four life stages: childhood, youthhood, adulthood and old age. They correspond respectively to *shao – yang*, *tai – yang*, *tai – yin* and *shao – yin* of the energy period.

Childhood is to the springtime of life when all species come back to life and are delicate by nature. It is the growth stage when the energy builds up. As the energy of the sky and the earth accumulates day by day, plants absorb and perceive the energy and the information of universe, beginning to change gradually. After sprouting, earring up and blooming, plants outgrow their weakness and thrive. In spring, vegetation mainly grows rather than bears fruit. Experiencing summer's luxuriance and autumn's maturation, the accumulation of energy inside the plant reaches its peak. Guided by the genetic information, the stored energy turns into ripe fruits, paving the way for the next period of life.

Children at puberty, just like budding plants in spring , is delicate and need to be fully protected both physically and mentally. By the law of the operation of energy in the four seasons, *Yellow Emperor's Classic of Medicine* makes the inference that what is born shouldn't be killed and what is given shouldn't be taken a-way.

The style of nurturing children is to give them enough encouragement and guidance to make them develop well, urging them to explore the unknown. Within safety, do not impose too many restrictions on them, otherwise the natural instincts of children may be destroyed. If children misbehave themselves, make sure to give them proper guidance. A warm and well – meant environment should be created to make children grow in a self – improving way and smoothly enter into the prom-ising youth. When educating children, radical punishment should be avoided, and too heavy a burden shouldn't be put on children mentally or physically.

Children's nature conforms to the characteristics of *Shao – yang*, therefore, we find children love praise and encouragement in daily life. The more children are praised, the better they behave. Conversely, harsh criticism or restrictions, or such devastating measures as threat and oppression adopted to make children yield to adults' will only destroy their *Shao – yang* Qi, resulting in illnesses and personality disorders.

Children haven't enter into the adult society, so it is not desirable to treat children as adults. In particular, we can't judge a child with adult values. Many great figures used to be regurded as retarded children when young. If someone re-quires a seedling fruit tree to bear fruit in spring, it is this person's fault rather than the tree. A great number of parents hold high hopes for their children, with the expectation that every aspect of their children meets their requirements and their children rank among the superior. Children should have good grades, be well mannered, in a word, everything children do should measure up to the norms. The expectation, requirement of children according to grown – ups' norms and values may seriously do harm to children's physical and mental health.

If *Qi* of *shao – yang* is damaged in childhood, it cannot make a normal shift to the aggressive, energetic stage of *tai – yang* when a person enters youth. As for the periodic operation of energy, if one stage is not completed, the next will be af-fected. Just as a late train, if it cannot make it to this station on time, then it can-not be punctual at the next. In this way, its journey ahead may be unpredictable.

Youthhood

Youthhood is equivalent to the summer of the year, that is, the energy of the earth surface received reaches the peak. As the intercourse between the sky Qi and the earth Qi is intense, vegetation thrive with luxuriant foliage, the cells inside the body metabolize vigorously, the exchanges of energy and information between man and the outside world reach the peak. Therefore, in youth, physical stamina, spirit, emotional and intellectual development are all at their peaks. No doubt, it is a period when one has the richest emotions and it's the best time to fall in love. Love is one of the most intense ways to exchange information, so love in youth will always remain in one's memory.

Summer and youthhood are a period of absorbing external energy and dispersing the internally stored energy in large quantities. Therefore, youth's behavior should adjust to this summer characteristic of life, receiving large amounts of the information from the outside world and enriching oneself by the exchange and collision of ideas. The lifestyle and behavior pattern should be focused on exchanging and screening out information, and thus, college rather than kindergarten or primary school, is the period when one's learning capacities are fully developed.

Young people prefer to participate in all kinds of activities but not to stay with their parents who used to take care of and put constraints on them, which is caused by the energy characteristic of $tai-yang$ phase. Mothers should not feel lost because your child has his or her own life, which indicates that your child starts to enter the summer of his or her life. Suppose your child depends on you as much as he or she used to in childhood in this stage, that will be a real trouble.

When it came to preserving health in summer, ancient Chinese scholars made an interesting analogy, stating that your favorite thing is left outdoors, so you always feel like going out instead of staying indoors, which is an outward reflection of the need for the energy inside your body to disperse rather than to store up. Partying, making friends, joining clubs, going on excursions, falling in love, etc. are all young people's favorite ways of socializing. If the process is purposefully restrained, then physical and mental problems may arise. The highest incidence rate of mental diseases among young people is related to the barrier to socializing and falling in love at this period. Therefore, the taboo for young people's love affair is to force the lovebirds to break up.

Without the adequate absorption in spring, there are no vigorous exchanges in summer. Lack of desire or drive to communicate with the outside world in youthhood originates from the shortage of spring Qi of $shao-yang$ in childhood. The otaku phenomenon in China stems from the restraints of childhood and adolescence schooling and improper parenting on Qi of $shao-yang$ of the children.

Trees cannot be heavily laden with fruits in autumn without the intense exchanges in summer. If the mission at any phase of $yin-yang$ of the four seasons fails to be accomplished, when the phase of maturation or storage comes, regrets in life cannot be avoided. Old life with regrets, means one cannot "die peacefully". For different stages of life, there are different tasks to be fulfilled. Every phase, inclusive of spring blossom and autumn fruit, has to obey the law of the operation of energy in the four seasons.

善言天者必验于人（二）
——生命在呼吸之间

The laws of the universe can be tested by human beings（Part Two）
——Life exists with breath

在中国古人的思想里，地球是有生命的，因为有生命，故能孕育万物。万物因地球能量有规律地运行和水的参与而生，所以万物的运行规律秉承了天地的运行规律，以及以水作为能量交流的介质这个特性。就好像母亲生出的孩子，必然带有母亲生命的基本特征。

虽然万物在形态上千差万别，但在基本的能量和信息层面，万物和天地遵从相同的规律，即生长收藏规律。中国古人在研究生长收藏规律时，使用了阴阳五行的理论模型。所以阴阳五行的理论体系既适用于研究天地之变，又适用于研究人体之变，故曰"善言天者，必有验于人"。

为研究天地能量运行规律而设计出来的数学模型，如果把它用之于人的生命研究，需要把阴阳、五行和代表生长收藏的太少阴阳对应于人体的组织结构和生理功能。在天人合一的背景下，建立人体的生命运动模型，这是中医基础理论的来源。

1. 生命在呼吸之间

天地之间能量的出入交汇赋予了地球生命，让她变成了一个富有生机的星球。在年周期里，春夏时节，从天而来的能量逐日增加，就好像此时天在呼出能量而大地在吸收从天而来的能量。到了秋冬时节，随太阳南移，变成了大地呼出以前吸收的能量，而天在吸入能量，地表空间在水的参与下，完成天地能量之间的交汇。这相当于天地呼吸的周期，人的呼吸类同于此。

在年周期里，随着太阳南移，大地可以呼出的能量越来越少，所以辐射到近地空间的能量也越来越少。随着地表空间的能量减少，温度越来越低，缺少能量时水分就不能蒸腾循环，所以空气越来越干燥。这就是秋冬时节的气候特征，一直到大地的呼出到了一个极点——"冬至"之后，太阳开始北移，天辐射到地球的能量增加，地面开始吸收能量，这是新一轮周期的开始。

地气上而为云，天气降而为雨，近地空间通过水循环完成了天地能量的交汇。人因天地合气而生，所以人的生命规律和运行方式是天地运行的全息缩小版。现代生理学的研究发现，人通过肺的外呼吸和细胞的内呼吸完成体内外能量的交换，这个交换是以人体的水循环为基础的。肺的呼吸运动，本身就可以作为人体能量交换和能量运行的代表，所以观察一个人的呼吸运动，就可以知道一个人的能量运行状态，从而推断出此人的健康状态。

在中医理论体系里，肺与外界相通。它与外界气体交换所获得的能量相当于人身之天气；脾胃消化吸收食物分解的水谷精微，上输于肺，相当于地气上升于天，肺从外界吸入的空气与脾上输于肺的精微物质在心中混合之后化生出营卫之气，这就是人体生命活动的基础物质——气血，这个肺气与脾气交汇产生新物质的过程，相当于天地氤氲化生万物的过程。

肺的呼吸运动，从外在的结果来看是吸入氧气和排出二氧化碳。吸是天气的下降，呼是地气的上临，在一呼一吸之间，身体内部进行了一系列的能量和物质的转化。这个反应的目的只有一个，就是通过呼吸，完成人体内部与外界环境之间物质能量的交换，俗称新陈代谢，而这个过程相当于天地之气交汇而孕育万物生命的过程，古人把这个过程叫做"氤氲化醇"。

2. 四气化六气

人的呼吸周期是这样的：呼气到了极点的时候有一个短暂的停顿，然后转入到吸气过程。在吸气刚刚开始的时候单位时间内吸气量比较少，吸气的过程越到后期，单位时间内的吸气量越大，接近极点时呼吸量达到最大值，这是一个自然呼吸的正常变化过程。我们把空气的进入看做外界能量的进入，称为"阳"，那么吸气量由少到多的过过渡就类似于四时阴阳中能量从少阳到太阳的生长过程。

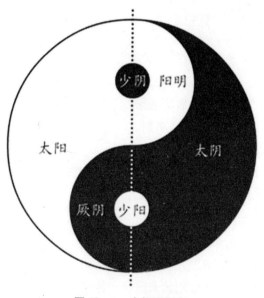

少阴 阳明

太阳

太阴

厥阴 少阳

图 18 - 1　太极阴阳图

吸气到了极点也会出现一个短暂的停顿，然后转入呼气阶段。呼气在刚刚开始的时候单位时间里呼出量最大，随着呼出过程的延长，单位时间内呼出量越来越少，直到呼出到了极点再次出现一个短暂的停顿。呼出可以看是做体内能量外出的代表，故呼气称之为"阴"，"阴"从强到弱，相当于四时阴阳中从太阴到少阴的过渡。

从一吸一呼可以看到人体能量的运行规律是从少阳到太阳，然后转入太阴到少阴结束，一个呼吸周期就代表了人体完成了一个能量交换。类似于以年为周期一个春夏秋冬的循环，代表了天地能量运行的周期，所以在中国有句古话叫"人体小天地，天地大人体"。

大家有没有发现在四时阴阳这个周期里，少阳－太阳到了极点之后，必须转到阴，而阴从太阴－少阴到了极点之后要转到阳？如果没有这个转折，就不能形成阴阳的周期变化。如果天地之间，阳不转阴，地面的温度就要无限制地升高；阴不转阳，地面温度就会无限制地降低。如果没有阴阳之间的停顿和转折，就形成不了地球的四时阴阳变化。转化期也是四时阴阳周期的两个阶段，这两个阶段加上太少阴阳四个阶段，一个生长收藏的周期里，就由六个阶段组成。

那么从阳转阴或者从阴转阳时，这个转折点的能量运行状态该如何描述呢？

我们已经知道能量的积累过程为少阳，能量的大进大出为太阳，能量的大量散发为太阴，能量的少量散发为少阴。在中医里，把能量从阳转到阴的这个阶段，称为阳明；把能量出到极点转入吸收的这个阶段，称为厥阴。"阳明"和"厥阴"加上少阳太阳与太阴少阴，六种能量流动过程，就构成了天地和人体的"能量"和"物质"的循环与交换。所以在中医理论里，人体完整的能量运行分为六个阶段：厥阴，少阳，太阳，阳明，太阴，少阴。

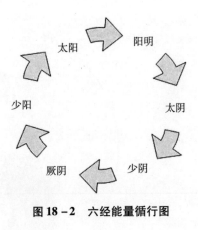

图18－2　六经能量循行图

如此一来，在少阳、太阳和太阴、少阴四时阴阳里增加了阳明与厥阴两种气，变为六气。六气运行构成了完整的四时阴阳周期。所以少阳、太阳、阳明、太阴、少阴、厥阴是天地之间也是人体生命六种基本的物质和能量运行轨道，这是中医理论里除阴阳之外，第二个基本理论模型。六气在人体生命理论模型里演变成了六经概念。如果六气中任何一个过程出现异常，就成为六经病变。这就是中医临床经典著作《伤寒论》的立论基础，俗称六经病。六气在人体对应于六经，六经各分手足（天地），化为人体的十二经络，这是人体经络模型的来源。

3. 呼吸运动与能量交换

提到呼吸我们最容易想到的是口鼻的呼吸。其实在生命体内部，还有一个更重要的呼吸，叫做内呼吸，即细胞和人体组织液与血管内血液进行物质交换，物质进入细胞内被分解代谢释放出能量，代谢废物通过一系列输转过程排出细胞外。内呼吸产生的能量被机体利用，这个吸收能源物质和排泄代谢产物可以概括为"入"和"出"两个阶段，这个过程的实质是能量的吸收和利用。所以内呼吸也有生长收藏四个阶段。内呼吸是人体生命的基础，也是新陈代谢的基本单位，一切疾病的产生都是新陈代谢的异常，也就是内呼吸的异常。

内呼吸和外呼吸在周期上是始终保持一致的，所以通过一个人外在的呼吸状态，就可以了解内呼吸的状态，从而推知其健康状态。呼吸周期如同一年中的四季变化，这个周期的完整代表了一年当中的风调雨顺。如果春不暖、夏不热、秋不凉、冬不寒，这叫"四时失序"。

古人认为人的"生命在呼吸之间"，一呼一吸，是一个能量运动的周期。那么一个人的呼吸如果浅快急促，说明这个人的阴阳周期异常，能量的生长收藏过程和物质的代谢周期异常。一个人的呼吸匀长和缓，就代表六气运行正常，阴阳周期完整，所以身体健康。

一个失去健康的成年人，他们的呼吸往往是浅快重浊的，浅快代表周期不完整，重浊是因为出入不充分。此类体质的人，他们细胞的内呼吸也存在同样的问题，即细胞质内积存了大量的废物排泄不出去，这种废物一是因过度摄入而没有被使用的营养物，二是未能排泄的代谢产物。这种堆积物阻碍了内呼吸的物质能量交换，所以细胞内呼吸和外在的呼吸运动一样，也维持在一个低水平的状态。如此一来，呼吸周期不完全，这个人的生命力就比较微弱，表现于外就是呼吸浅快粗重。因为细胞能量代谢不完全，不但身体各项机能不足，同时也表现在抗病修复能力和免疫能力的不足。所以观察一个人的呼吸，就可以知道身体各部位的机能状态，包括抗压抗病能力，运动生殖能力等。

肥胖症患者的肺部和组织细胞以及组织间隙内堆积了大量的代谢垃

圾，影响了肺和细胞的内外呼吸，所以呼吸短促。遇到剧烈运动需要大量能量支持的时候，就会感觉气息不够、体力不支。这说明内部能量运行不健，也就是六气运行不健。六气运行不健对身体的影响是全方位的，所以只要有肥胖症，同时就会伴有心脏、关节、骨骼和性功能等多系统疾病，女性肥胖症患者还会伴有月经疾病和不育症。

在生活中我们也有这种经验，同等条件下，呼吸浅快的人健康状况较呼吸平稳绵长的人差，不但体能较弱而且各项生理功能相对都比较低下。大家观察熟睡中的小孩，就可以体会呼吸均匀绵长是一种什么状态，好像在用腹部呼吸，每一次呼和吸都能达到极点，吸入和呼出的过程都比较长，这代表良好的新陈代谢。而呼吸浅快最有代表性的是临终前的呼吸状态，短而急促，呼吸深度几乎就在嗓子附近徘徊，是气机的升降沉浮和生命生长收藏周期将要完结的先兆。所以对普通人来说，当你自己觉得呼吸时气息不够，容易喘息疲劳的时候，就代表身体的生命机能在下降。

说到呼吸，其实大多数人的呼吸都是不充分的，在安逸的生活条件下，没有体力活动，人的呼和吸就不能到达极点。长此以往，呼吸的幅度会越来越小，影响了精微物质和代谢产物的出入，这是造成呼吸浅快的原因之一。体育锻炼可以令呼吸深度加大，在呼出和吸入的两端达到极点，如此一来，组织细胞生长收藏四个阶段都会达到极致，这就是运动可以保持身体健康的原因。

假如一个人肺活量小，就意味着能量摄入和吸收的不足。婴儿出生时，如果哭声大，爷爷奶奶会就喜形于色，因为响亮持久的哭声代表了身体内部能量周期处于健康的状态。

呼吸代表了人体能量物质的交换和四时阴阳的运行周期，那么观察一个人的呼吸深度和频率，就可以知道他的健康状况。不仅如此，中医大夫，通过观察一个人呼吸的幅度、频率以及伴随症状，可以了解到一个人身体的病因以及病情的深度，推知出很多生活和身体的信息。对不了解中医的人来说，这个过程会显得非常神奇，其实这套技术是中医诊断疾病的基本功。不仅如此，中医理论体系里，有一套"五行"理论，通过一个人身体外在的表现可以推断出身体内部的运行状态和病变部位以及病变原因，这就是中医里的"望闻问切"诊断方法。这种诊断方法的设计原理出自阴阳五行和六气学说，通过外在现象推知体内阴阳变化，所以《黄帝内经》里说"谨熟阴阳，无与众谋"。

In the ancient Chinese mind, the earth is alive. The earth has a life, so it breeds all species. All species are born because of the regular evolution of energy of the earth and the participation of water. Therefore, the operation of all species naturally obeys the law of nature with water as the medium of energy exchange. Just like a mother's child, it must have the basic characteristics of a mother's life.

Through the vast difference in the forms of all species, all species and the nature must follow the same law of energy and information, namely the law of "growth, flourish maturation and storage". When ancient Chinese studied the law of"growth, flourish maturation and storage", they used the theoretical models of "*Yin* and *Yang*" and the " *five phases*". Therefore, the theory of *Yin Yang* and *five phases* is suitable not only for studying the changes of the universe, but also for human body. Accordingly, it is said "the laws of the universe can be tested by human beings. "

The mathematical model was designed to study the law of energy transformation in the universe. If adopt it to study human life, the concepts of *Yin Yang*, the *five phases* and the *Tai Shao Yin Yang* (greater/lesser Yin Yang) need to conform to the organizational structure and physiological functions of human body. The human life model should be built under the principle of harmony between man and the universe, which is the source of the basic theory of traditional Chinese medicine.

1. Life exists with breath

The interaction of energy between the sky and the earth gives lives of all species on the earth, making her a living planet. In one year period, the energy from the sky increases every day during spring and summer, as if the sky exhales the energy while the earth inhales the energy from the sky. In autumn and winter, with the sun moving to the south, this process has become that the earth exhales previously absorbed energy while the sky inhales the energy. The terrestrial space completes the interaction of the energy between the sky and the earth with the participation of water. This one year's process am be reffered to as the respiration of the nature. And meanwhile, a human's respiration is similar to this.

In one year period, after the summer solstice, the earth exhales the energy less with the sun moving to the south, so the radiation to the terrestrial space reduces. As the irradiated energy to the terrestrial space decreases, the temperature gets lower, and thus the hydrological cycle runs ineffectively, and the air gets drier. This is the climate characteristic of autumn and winter. This process continues until the exhaling of the earth reaches an end——called "winter solstice". And then the sun begins to move northward. The sky exhales the energy increasingly while the earth inhales the energy. This is the beginning of a new period.

The earth – Qi rises and becomes cloud while the sky – Qi falls and becomes rain. The interaction of energy between the sky and the earth is thus completed by the hydrological cycle in the terrestrial space. Man is born in intercourse of the earth – Qi and the sky – Qi. Therefore, the law of human life and its evolution mode is the exact holographic edition of the universe. Modern physiological studies have found that people perform the internal and external energy exchange through the external respiration of the lung and intracellular respiration of the cells. This exchange is based on the fluid circulation of the human body. The respiration of the lungs can act as a proxy for the energy exchange and evolution of the body. That is to say, we can roughly infer a person's health status only by observing his breath. That's why we can diagnose a patient quickly and accurately.

In the theoretical system of TCM, the lungs interlink with the outside world, and the energy, obtained by exchanging with the outside Qi, is equivalent to the "Tian Qi"(sky – Qi) of the human body. Essence of water and food, which are digested by stomach and absorbed by the spleen, moves up to the lungs. This process is equivalent to rising "earth – Qi" to the sky. The air absorbed by the lungs from the outside is mixed with the essence of water and food that moved from the spleen to the lungs. And then it gives birth to the "Qi of Ying Wei", which is the basic matter of human life activity – "Qi and blood". The interaction process between the lung – Qi and spleen – Qi produces a new matter, corresponds to the process of that all species on the earth are created by "earth – Qi" and "sky – Qi".

The respiration of the lungs, from their external manifestation, is a process of the inhalation of oxygen and the exhaling of carbon dioxide. The inhalation is the descent of the "sky – Qi" while the exhalation is the rise of the "earth – Qi". In one breath period, there is a series of transformations of energy and matter within the body. The only purpose of this reaction is to complete the exchange of the material and energy between the human body and the external environment through breathing. It is commonly called metabolism. This process corresponds to the process of that all species on the earth are created by "earth – Qi" and "sky – Qi". The ancient Chinese called this process "Yingyun Huachun".

2. Four Qi transfers into six Qi

One respiratory period of human is like this process: when the exhalation reaches its peak, there will be a short pause and then it turns into the inhalation process. At the beginning of inhalation, the inhalation quantity is less in unit time. The inspiratory capacity grows with the inhalation process prolongs, untill the maximum respiration quantity. This is a normal process of natural respiration. If the entry of air is considered as that of the external energy, called "Yang", then the suction volume increases, which is similar to the increasing process of the energy from *Shaoyang* to *Taiyang* in the "*Si – shi Yin Yang*" (four stages of Yin – yang: grath, flourish maturation and storage) model.

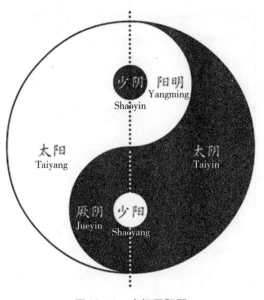

图 18 – 1　太极阴阳图

When the inhalation reaches its peak, there will be a short pause, too, and then it transfers to the exhalation process. At the beginning of the exhalation, the expiratory volume in unit time is the maximum, with the expiration extending, the exhaled volume per unit time decreases until the exhalation reaches its peak a-gain, together with a short pause. The exhalation process can be considered as an output of energy from the body, so the exhalation called "*Yin*". "*Yin*" changes from strong to the weak, equivalent to the process from *Tai − yin* to *Shao − yin* in the "*Si − shi Yin Yang*"model.

In one respiratory cycle, the energy of the human body runs from *Shao − yang* to *Tai − yang*, and then from *Tai − yin* to *Shao − yin*, that is, the completion of an energy exchange for the human body. Similar to the period of spring, sum-mer, autumn and winter in one year, it represents the cycle of the energy of the u-niverse. Therefore, there is an old Chinese saying, "the human body is a small u-niverse, and the universe is a large human body. "

Have you found that, in one cycle of *Si − shi Yin Yang*, it must turn to *Yin* when *Tai − Yang* reaches its peak, while it must turn back to Yang when *Shao − yin* reaches its peak. Without this transition, the periodical change of *Yin* and *Yang* would not be formed. If *Yang* does not transfer to *Yin* between the earth and the sky, the temperature of the ground will increase without limit. By the same way, if the *Yin* does not transfer to *Yang*, the temperature of the ground will be lowered without limit. Without the pauses and transitions between *Yin* and *Yang*, there is no change in the *Si − shi Yin Yang* of the earth. The two transition periods are also included in the *Si − shi Yin Yang* cycle. These two periods, together with *Shao − yang*, *Tai − yang*, *Tai − yin* and *Shao − yin*, are the six stages in one cycle of "growth, flourish maturation and storage".

Then how to describe the energy operation status of these two transformation stages from *Yang* to *Yin* or from *Yin* to *Yang*?

We have already known that the accumulation process of energy is *Shao − yang*, the process of the greater energy input and output is *Tai − yang*, the mas-sive dissipation of energy is *Tai − yin*, and the small dissipation of energy is *Shao − yin*. In TCM, the stage of transferring energy from *Yang* to *Yin* is called *Yang − ming*. The stage for the energy changing the output to the absorption is called *Jueyin. Yang − ming* and *Jue − yin*, together with *Shao − yang*, *Tai − Yang*, *Tai − yin* and *Shao − yin* are six kinds of energy flowing processes, which make up the circulation and exchange of energy and matter between the universe and the human body. Therefore, the whole period of energy circulation in body is consisted of six stages: *Jue – yin, Shao – yang, Tai – yang, Yang – ming, Tai – yin* and *Shao – yin*.

In this way, *Yangming* and *Jueyin* are added to the *Si – shi Yin Yang* process, and it becomes six Qi. The regular operation of six Qi constitutes a complete *Si – shi Yin Yang* cycle. Therefore, *Shao – yang, Tai – yang, Yang –*

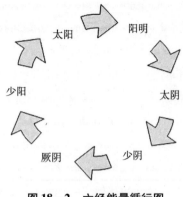

图 18 – 2 六经能量循行图

ming, Tai – yin, Shao – yin and *Jue – yin* are the six basic matters and also energy operation tracks within the universe and human body. This is the second basic theoretical model in TCM theory except "*Yin Yang*". Six Qi in the human life theory model has evolved into the concepts of six meridians. If six Qi is abnormal, a six – meridian lesion, commonly known as the sixmeridian disease, will happen. This is the theoretical foundation of *Treatise on Cold Damage and Miscellaneous Diseases*, a clinical classic of TCM. Six Qi in the body corresponds to six meridians. Six meridians are separated and correspond to hands and feet (that is similar to the sky and the earth). Accordingly, there are 12 meridians in the human body, which is the origin of the body meridian model.

3. Respiration and energy exchange

When it comes to respiration, the first thing occurs is the breathing by mouth and nose. In fact, there is a more important breath within a living body, called internal breathing. The cells and tissue fluid of the human body carries out material exchange with blood in vessels, and the material enters the cells and is released into energy by catabolism, and the waste is excreted through a series of transportation processes. The energy produced by the internal respiration is utilized by the organs. This absorption of energy and metabolite of excretion can be summed up as two stages: "input" and "output", respectively. The essence of this process is the absorption and utilization of energy. So internal breathing also has four stages of "growth, flourish maturation and storage". Internal breathing is not only the basis of human life, but also the basic unit of metabolism. All diseases are caused by abnormal metabolism, that is, the abnormal internal breathing.

Internal breathing and external breathing share a same period. So internal breathing state can be inferred by external breathing state, and so do the health condition. One respiration period is like the four seasons of a year. The complete period represents that the wind and rain come in their time in a year. When spring is not warm, summer is not hot, autumn is not cool, winter is not cold, any one of them occurs could be called"Si – shi disordered"(disorder of four seasons).

The ancient Chinese believed that human life existed in respiration. Every respiration is a period of energy operation. If A person's breath is shallow and rapid, the period of his/her *Yin* and *Yang* is abnormal, the energy process of"birth, growth, flourish maturation and storage"and the metabolic period of material is abnormal. If a person's breathing is long and slow, it means the six Qi runs normally, the *Yin – Yang* period is complete, and the body is healthy.

An unhealthy adult, his respiration is often shallow – fast or deep – muddy. Shallow – fast indicates the incomplete cycle. Deep – muddy is due to inadequate inhalation and exhalation. People with this kind of constitution also have the same problems of internal respiration in their cells. That is, a large amount of waste is stored in the cytoplasm and can not be excreted. The waste contents nutrient that is excessively consumed by the cell but not used, and the metabolite that fails to excrete. This accumulation impedes the exchange of material and energy within internal respiration. Therefore, the intracellular respiration, the same as the external respiration, maintains at a low level. As a result, the respiration period is incomplete, and the vitality of this person is relatively weak. The outer manifestation is that his breathing is often shallow – fast or deep – muddy. Because the cellular energy metabolism is not complete, the body functions are not only insufficient, but also manifested the insufficiency in the repair ability and the immunity ability against diseases . Accordingly, by observing a person's respiration, one can know the health status of various parts of the body, including pressure tolerance, disease resistance, exercising functions, reproductive ability, and so on.

For obese patients, large amounts of metabolic wastes are accumulated in the cells of their lungs and tissues, as well as in the tissue spaces. These metabolic wastes interfere with the internal and external respirations of lungs and cells, resulting in shallow – fast breathing. When they have strenuous exercises that require a lot of energy, they will feel shallow – fast breathing and physical weaknesses. This shows that the internal energy is not healthy, that is, the operation of the six Qi is not in the right tracks. The unhealthy operations of the six Qi affect negatively the body in all aspects. Therefore, as long as there is obesity, there will be also many systemic diseases in heart, joints, bones and sexual functions. Obese women would also suffer from menstrual diseases and infertility.

We have also this experience in daily life, that people who breathe shallow – fast are in poorer health than those who breathe long – smoothly under the same conditions. They are not only physically weak, but also have relatively low physiological functions. When you observe one sleeping child, you can understand what kind of breathing state is evenly – long lasting. He seems to breathe through the belly. Every breath can reach its peak. They inhale and exhale for a long period of time, which represents good metabolism. The most typical shallow fast breathing state happened before death, short and rapid, and the breathing almost hovers around the throat. This is a bad omen of that the operation of the Qi and the life span will be over. For the ordinary people, therefore, when you feel your breath not enough, and easy to be tired in breathing, it means that your functions are declining.

When it comes to respiration, most people's respiration is not sufficient. In a comfortable living condition, one's exhalation and inhalation can't reach the maximun without physical activities. Over time, the amplitude of respiration will become smaller and smaller, affecting the exchange of essence materials and metabolites. This is one of the causes of shallow – fast breathing. Physical exercises can increase the amplitude of breathing, reaching the maximum at both exhalation and inhalation. As a result, the"growth, flourish maturation and storage"four stages of tissue cells will reach the perfection. That's why exercises can keep fit.

If a person's lung capacity is small, it means lack of energy intake and absorption. When a baby is born, his grandparents will be happy if he cries loudly. Because a loud and persistent cry represents a healthy state of energy period within his body.

Since the respiration represents the exchange period of energy and materials and the operation period of Si – shi Yin Yang, one can infer the amplitude and frequency of a person's breath to know his health condition. More than this, TCM doctors can judge the cause and the disease severity of one patient and deduce out a lot of his life and physical information by observing the amplitude and frequency of breath and associated symptoms. For those who do not understand TCM, the diagnosis process will be very magical. In fact, this set of diagnosis technique is the basic skill for TCM doctors in diagnosing diseases. Moreover, there is a set of "*five phases*" theory in the TCM system. The theory of "*five phases*" can infer the internal operation state of the body, the location of the lesion and the cause of the diseases through the outer manifestation of a person's body. This is the basic diagnosis method in the traditional Chinese medicine, that is, *look, listen, question* and *feel the pulse*. The principle of this diagnostic method is derived from the theory of "*Yin Yang*", "*five phases*" and "*six Qi*". One can infer changes of *Yin* and *Yang* in the human body by external manifestations. Therefore, as said in *Yellow Emperor's Classic of Medicine*, you don't have to consult with the others if you can skillfully use the theory of *Yin Yang*.

五行藏象论

Visceral manifestation theory by the Five Phases

一方水土养一方人

人体随时随地与外界环境进行着能量交换，并且依赖从外界环境中获取的能量而生存。那么，外界环境的能量种类、数量、结构以及能量形式对生命体的能量运行就有着举足轻重的影响。自古以来，人类逐水草而居就是为了选择在最好的能量环境下繁衍生息。

人体从外界获取能量的方式和途径多种多样，包括肺与皮肤的呼吸，眼耳鼻舌各种感官获得的感受。这些能量有些是有形可见的，有些是无形不可见的。比如阳光、声音甚至耳朵不能感知的声波，都是能量存在的方式。在所有人体必需的能量形式中，最常见的能量存在方式是食物。物质是能量存在方式之一种。人类通过对食物的摄取、消化和吸收，把食物包含的能量转化为人体所需要的能量，供给身体使用，以完成四时阴阳周期变化下生生不息的生命新陈代谢。食物中包含的能量特性，或生发或收藏之气，被身体吸收后，身体就会产生相应的能量特性，所以长期吃生发之力比较旺盛食物的人，身体能量运行也就有了生发旺盛的能量特点。

人生活环境中存在的阳光、空气、色彩、声音、气味、形态、情绪等一切外界事物，组成生命存在的外部环境。因为这些元素都是能量和信息体，它们组合成了一个能量和信息场。人生活在这个能量信息场中，通过感觉器官以及意识活动与外界能量信息场进行交换，所以外界环境的能量信息特点就决定了人体内部能量的特点。也就是说外在的环境因素在影响人体内部能量的运行，这是中医里人体内环境与外环境"同气相求，同频共振"的规律。

不同的环境有不同的能量以及信息场。人们长期在某个区域内生活，久而久之就带上了这个地域的能量和信息特征。一方水土养一方人，就是外界能量信息场对人体内部能量信息场的作用而形成的人伦现象。

在生活中我们会发现，美味可口的饮食，会令人周身舒泰，心情愉悦。如果食物质量低劣或使用过量添加剂，吃过之后不仅身体不适而且容易产生消沉甚至狂暴的负面情绪。这是因为食物分解之后，包含在物质当中的能量信息被还原出来之后，这种能量结构是否纯正、和谐，直接影响到人体的能量运行周期。不同品质的食物会引起不同的身心反应以及能量运行方式，所以中国人在饮食上讲究五味调和，就是为了使人体获得的能量更符合身体内部四时阴阳周期的平衡。那么"五味调和"和"能量运行"有什么关系呢？

五行的来历

中国人认为"气聚而成形，形散而化气"，物质和能量本为一体，只是表现形式不同。"气"指的是能量的运动，"形"指的是可见的物质，物质可以看做是能量的一种储存方式。人类最早是利用自身的感觉器官，通过认识物理现象来认识世界，后来又发明了仪器来认识超越人感觉器官的能量存在方式。古人没有现代化的仪器，所以他们认识世界采取了取象比类的方式来认识物质背后的能量属性。

事物之间的相互影响是通过能量相互作用来完成的，所以要研究事物之间以及人与外界之间的能量作用，可以忽略掉物质形态方面的差异，只从它所包含的能量属性上来认识事物。假如知道了一种食物的能量属性，当我们需要某种属性的能量时，只要吃带有这种能量属性的食物就可以达到目的。同样我们需要某种信息属性时，只要从感官上设置一个带有这种信息属性的场就可以做到。每个女孩在约会的时候，都会穿上最美丽的衣裳，这就是人类对能量信息的使用。

事物的能量的周期分为生长收藏四个阶段，一年当中春夏秋冬的物候变化最能反映四种能量的特征。古人根据阴阳出入的变化，把一个能量运行周期分为四个阶段，称为"太少阴阳"。但是太少阴阳四种变化是在无形的能量运行层面上规定的，是无形不可见的。一年当中四时阴阳消长引起物候变化，我们通过莺飞草长、大雁北归这些现象才能意识到其能量的改变。所以对能量的划分，除了四气之外，在有形的物质世界里，还需要一种方法来判定有形物质之中包含的能量属性，这种能量在物质成型的阶段，可以认为是固化的，当物质分解之后，才能释放出自己的能量。

我们知道天地能量的变化是无形的，四气能量运行要作用于大地，引起水土的变化，进而产生动植物种种生命现象。而春、夏、秋、冬分别对应于"木""火""金""水"。还有一种主管氤氲变化的能量，名之为"土"。加上"木火金水"，世间共有五种基本的能量"存在"形式，就是"木火土金水"。

注意"木火土金水"是能量的存在方式，而不是能量的运行方式，运行方式是少阳、太阳、太阴、少阴加上阳明和厥阴六种方式，称为"六气"。

在中国古人眼里，代表生发之力的木，代表发散之力的火，代表下降之力的金，代表收藏之力的水，以及代表转化之力的土，是组成世界的五种基本能量元素。这里的木火土金水，并不是实指的树木、火焰、或者石头，而是以可感受到的物质，来指代不可见的能量特性，这就是"取象比类"的意思。只要带有生发特性的事物，我们都可以认为其带有"木"的特性，就好像少年儿童有蓬勃朝气，我们就说这是人生的春天。

五季与五行的能量及生化特性列表：

春发生之纪（木），是谓启陈。生气淳化，万物以荣。

夏赫曦之纪（火），是谓蕃茂。天地气交，万物华实。

暑敦阜之纪（土），是谓广化。顺长以盈，物化充成。

秋坚成之纪（金），是谓收引。秋高气爽，物以司成。

冬流衍之纪（水），是谓封藏。天地严凝，水冰地坼。

五行关系

在一个生命系统内部，"木火土金水"五种能量形式有一个生克耗助泄的关系，简单的表达为木生火，火生土，土生金，金生水，水生木，金克木，木克土，土克水，水克火，火克金。系统通过这种关系的运动来调整维持内部的能量运行。故"木火土金水"被称为五行，"行"为运动之意，利用五行观点来认识和改变事物，就叫做"五行之法"，这是中医理论体系里的一个基本原理。

五行平衡是能量周期正常运行的基本条件。任何一方的不足或者过盛，首先通过内部的生克耗助泄关系来维持的，当内部的调整已经不足以纠偏时，就需要改善外部的能量输入来纠偏。那么来自外部的能量应该选择呢？中国古人把万事万物在不同层次做了五行归类。作为中医基础知识的介绍，我们把最简单的五行划分法归纳为下面的表格：

五音	五味	五色	五化	五气	五方	五季	五行	五脏	五腑	五官	形体	五液	五志	五声
角	酸	青	生	风	东	春	木	肝	胆	目	筋	泪	怒	呼
徵	辛	白	收	燥	西	秋	金	肺	大肠	鼻	皮	涕	悲	哭
宫	甘	黄	化	湿	中	长夏	土	脾	胃	口	肉	涎	思	歌
商	苦	赤	长	暑	南	夏	火	心	小肠	舌	脉	汗	喜	笑
羽	咸	黑	藏	寒	北	冬	水	肾	膀胱	耳	骨	唾	恐	呻

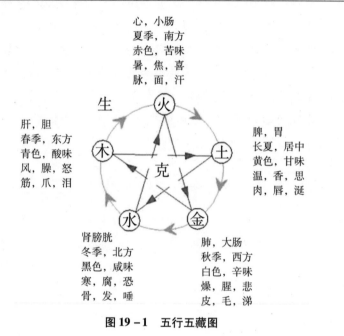

图 19–1　五行五藏图

对物质世界有了五行的划分，就可以掌握其能量属性，建立外在的能量场以调整身体内部的五行平衡和能量运行，这就是中医治病的原理。

五藏

五行能量在事物系统内的相互作用维持了系统的能量周期运行，我们把这个系统命名为太极。太极的运行是以五行之间的生克耗助泄来维持平衡，做为物质形式存在的人，也必有物质体来完成五行的功能，这个物质体就是中医里的"心火、肝木、脾土、肺金、肾水"五藏系统。

中医里的五藏系统既有实体的组织脏腑与之对应，同时五藏又是一个虚拟的功能概念。六气是系统内能量的运动过程，五行是系统内能量运行的阶段，所以它们在人体是可以统一起来的。古典中医里把五藏系统和六气结合在一起，划分了人体少阳相火、太阳寒水、少阴君火、太阴湿土、阳明燥金和厥阴风木六大系统。六大系统里各有主管能量运行和物质代谢的两个部分，合起来就是十二个子系统，以十二经来冠名，就是：

足少阳胆经、足太阳膀胱经、足阳明胃经、足太阴脾经、足少阴肾经、足厥阴肝经；手少阳三焦经、手太阳小肠经、手阳明大肠经、手太阴肺经、手少阴心经、手厥阴心包经。

十二经络是为了研究生命现象设计的虚拟概念，同时在人体又有相应的区间和脏腑与之对应，这就是中医里经络脏腑理论的来源。十二经络在人体内连脏腑，外连肢节，共同完成人体的物质代谢和能量交换。所以从十二经以及脏腑的病理改变，就可以推知人体内六气以及五脏五行的异常，从而选择相应的能量载体给予纠正。

Each place nurtures its own inhabitants

Human body exchanges energy with the environment whenever and wherever possible, and survives on the energy obtained from the environment. Then, the type, quantity, structure and form of the energy in the external environment would have a significant influence on the energy circulation of a living body. Since ancient times, humans have been living where there is water and grasses, just for the purpose of selecting the best energy environment to survive and multiply.

The human body gets the energy from the outside world in various ways, including respiration of the lungs and the skin and the perception of various tactile organs, such as eyes, ears, nose, tongue, and so on. Some of these energy are visible, while others invisible. For example, the sunlight, sound, and even the unperceived sound are existence states of energy. Among all the energies which the body needs, the most common form is food. Through the intake, digestion and absorption of food, the human body transfers the food energy to the energy that can be put to use by the body, and to complete the endless life metabolism, in accordance with the periodical changes of *Yin* and *Yang* of life in the four seasons. Since food contains its own energy characteristics, such as *Qi* of growth, or dormancy, it is inherited to the body when the food is eaten. Therefore, people who have a lot of vigorous food in the long term would be very energetic.

The external environment in which people live is usually composed of these items including the sunlight, air, color, sound and smell, etc. All these items are carriers of both energy and information, and thus form a field containing these energy and information. Human lives in this field, and he exchanges the energy and information with those of the outside world through the sense organs and consciousness activity. Therefore, the energy and information characteristics of the external environment decide that inside the human body. That is to say, the external environmental factors influence the internal energy operation of human body. This is exactly the law of"the same Qi absorbs each other and the same frequency resonates between the external and internal body environment"described in TCM.

五行藏象论

Different environments have different fields of energy and information. If people live in a certain area for a long time, then the energy and information features of this region will be taken by them. As an old Chinese saying goes, each place nurtures its own inhabitants, that is, the unique features of a local environment always give special characteristics to its inhabitants. That the external energy and information field plays a role in that of the human body is embodied in human relations.

We find that a delicious diet can make people feel happy and cheerful in daily life. If the food is poor in quality or over – processed by additives, one will not only feel uncomfortable, but he will also be prone to have negative emotions of depression and even rage after eating them. This is due to the fact that the energy and information of the eaten food is reproduced in the human body. The fact whether the characteristics of energy and information of food are pure and harmonious or not affects the energy operation of the human body directly. Different quality of food can give rise to different physical and mental reactions as well as different energy operation modes. Therefore, the Chinese people pay much attention to the harmony of"five flavors"in the diet in order to make the energy gained by the human body more in accordance with the balance between *Yin* and *Yang* of the body in the four periods. Then, what is the relationship between"five harmonized flavors"and"energy operation"?

The origin of *Five Phases*

Chinese people think that"the aggregation of *Qi* can transform into matter, and the disappearance of matter can transform into *Qi*(energy) ". Matter and energy are in essence an integral whole, but in different forms. *Qi* refers to the energy and its movement, and"*Xing*"refers to visible matter. Matter can be thought of as a form of energy storage. Human beings first used their sense organs to understand the world by recognizing physical phenomena. Later, scientific instruments were invented to help them recognize the existence of energy beyond human perception. The ancient Chinese did not have modern instruments, so they understood the world by recognizingthe energy attributes behind matter using analogy methodology.

The interaction among all things is accomplished by the interaction of energy. Therefore, to study the energy interaction among all things or between people and the surrounding environment, we can ignore the difference in the forms of matters, but recognize things only from the energy attributes it contains. Assuming we know the energy attribute of a kind of food, if we need energy of a specific attribute, we can eat the food with this kind of energy attribute to obtain it. Similarly, when we need some specific information attribute, we can set up a sense field with this kind of information attribute. For example, girls will wear the most beautiful clothes when she has a date. This is exactly a proper use of energy and information.

The energy period of matter is divided into four stages: growth, flourish maturation and storage. The phenological changes in spring, summer, autumn and winter of one year can directly reflect the characteristics of these four kinds of energy transformations. According to the changes of *Yin* and *Yang*, the ancient Chinese divided an energy operation period into four stages, called *"Tai Shao Yin Yang"*, that is, *Tai – Yin*(greater yin) , *Shao – Yin*(lesser yin) , *Shao – Yang*(lesser yang) and *Tai – Yang*(greater yang) . But the four changes in*"Tai Shao Yin Yang"*are defined on the invisible energy level, intangible and invisible. As for the phenological changes in a year caused by the growth and the decline of *Yin* and *Yang* in the four periods, we can recognize the change of energy by the phenomena of the grass growth and orioles chirping or wild geese migrating to the north. For the classification of energy in the tangible physical world, therefore, it needs a method, besides the four Qi, to determine the energy attributes of tangible matter. This energy is solidly fixed in the tangible matter, and will be released when the matter is decomposed and dissipated.

As we know, the energy change between the sky and the earth is invisible, and four Qi energy runs to act on the earth, causing the change of earth and water, and then resulting in a variety of life phenomena of animals and plants. The energy of spring , summer, autumn and winter correspond with wood , fire, metal and water respectively. There is another kind of energy, called "earth", in charge of all series of transformation. There are five basic existence forms of ener-

五行藏象论

gy, that is, "wood, fire, earth, metal and water". Please note that the "wood, fire, earth, metal and water" are the existence forms of energy, not their operation modes. The operation modes of five kinds of energy are *Shao – yang, Tai – yang, Tai – yin, Shao – yin,* and *Jue – yin* and *Yang – ming* called"six Qi".

For ancient Chinese, wood has germinal power, fire has dispersing power, metal has the declining power, water has storage power, and earth has transformation power. They are called the *Five Phases*, the five basic elements of energy that constitute the universe. The *Five Phases*, wood, fire, earth, metal and water mentioned here, are not real trees, flames, or stones, etc, but the invisible energy existences of matter that can be felt. This is what the analogy methodology means. For a thing with germinal characteristic, we can consider it as"wood"; just as a child is vigorous and energetic, we say this is the spring of his life.

Here we list the energy characteristics of five seasons and *five phases* and their features of engendering transformation:

Spring(wood), is called "Qichen". All nourished species are born and grow up.

Summer(fire), is called "Fanmao". Harmonious intercourse of the Sky – Qi and the Earth – Qi makes all vegetations on the earth blossom and preparing for bearing fruit.

Hot summer(earth), is called "Guanghua". All vegetations attend to the ripening of fruits.

Autumn(metal), is called"Shouyin". Autumn is cool with a clear sky. All vegetations mature.

Winter(water), is called"Fengcang". It is cold and freezing. All vegetations wither, entering into a dormancy state.

Relationship among the *five phases*

Within a living system, the five energies of"wood, fire, earth, metal and water"form an engendering or restraining relationship. To put it simply, wood engenders fire, fire engenders earth, earth engenders metal, metal engenders water, and water engenders wood. In contrast, metal restrains wood, wood restrains earth,

earth restrains water, water restrains fire and fire restrains metal. The living system adjusts and maintains the internal energy movement by the movement of *Five Phases*. Taking the perspective of five phases to know and change things is called "the *five phases* theory", which is a basic principle in the theoretical system of traditional Chinese medicine.

The balance among the five phases is the basic prerequisites for the normal operation of energy cycle. The deficiency or excess of any phase will firstly be adjusted by the internal engendering or restraining relations. When the internal adjustment is not sufficient enough to solve this problem, it is necessary to improve the external energy input to rectify the deviation. How to choose the external energy? The ancient Chinese classified everything by the five phases theory at different levels. As an introduction to the ABC of traditional Chinese medicine, we list the simplest division of the five phases in the following table:

five notes	Jue	Zhi	Gong	Shang	Yu
five tastes	sour	spicy	sweet	bitter	salty
five colours	cyan	white	yellow	red	black
five transformations	birth	degradation	transformation	growth	storage
five movements	wind	dryness	dampness	Summer heat	cold
five directions	east	west	center	south	north
five seasons	spring	autumn	long summer	summer	winter
five phases	wood	metal	earth	fire	water
five viscera	liver	lung	spleen	heart	kidney
five bowels	gallbladder	large intestine	stomach	small intestine	bladder
five sense organs		nose	mouth	tongue	ear
body		skin	muscle	vessel	bone
five fluids	tears	snivel	drool	sweat	spittle
five emotions	anger	sadness	anxiety	joy	fear
five voices	shout	cry	sing	laugh	groan

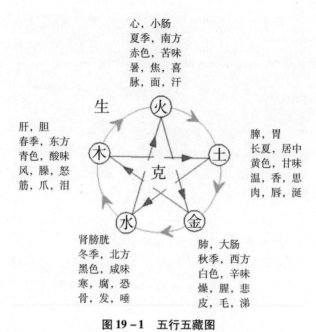

心，小肠
夏季，南方
赤色，苦味
暑，焦，喜
脉，面，汗

生

火

肝，胆
春季，东方
青色，酸味
风，臊，怒
筋，爪，泪

木

克

土

脾，胃
长夏，居中
黄色，甘味
温，香，思
肉，唇，涎

水

金

肾膀胱
冬季，北方
黑色，咸味
寒，腐，恐
骨，发，唾

肺，大肠
秋季，西方
白色，辛味
燥，腥，悲
皮，毛，涕

图 19 - 1　五行五藏图

Since the physical world is classified by the five phases theory, its energy attributes can be mastered, and the external energy field can be established to adjust the balance of five phases and energy movement within the body. This is the principle of treating diseases by traditional Chinese medicine.

Five – zang temples

The interaction of energy among the *five phases* in a system maintains its periodical movement of energy, and we call this system *Tai Ji*. The movement of *Tai Ji* is to maintain a balance among the *five phases* by their relations of engendering and restraining. A person must have the body to perform the functions of the five phases. From the viewpoint of traditional Chinese medicine, this body system is the five – zang temples system, that is, "heart temple(fire), liver temple(wood), spleen temple(earth), lung temple(metal) and kidney temple(water)".

In the traditional Chinese medicine, the five – zang temples system not only has physical viscera, but also is a virtual concept of energy at the same time. Six

Qi is the movement process of energy in the body system, and the five phases are the stages of energy operation in the system, so they can be unified in human body. In classical Chinese medicine the five – zang temples system and six Qi are integrated together. The human body is divided into six sub – systems: *Shao – yang*(ministerial fire) , *Tai – yang*(cold water) , *Shao – yin*(monarch fire) , *Tai – yin*(damp earth) , *Yang – ming*(dry metal) and *Jue – yin*(wind wood) . In each sub – system, there are two parts in charge of energy operation and food metabolism, and thus one body has 12 sub – systems in total, which are named after the 12 meridians. They are the Gallbladder Meridian of Foot – Shaoyang, the Bladder Meridian of Foot – taiyang, the Stomach Meridian of Foot – Yangming, the Spleen Meridian of Foot – Taiyin, the Kidney Meridian of Foot – Shaoyin, the Liver Meridian of Foot – Jueyin, the Triple Energizer Meridian of Hand – Shaoyang, the Small Intestine Meridian of Hand – taiyang, the Large Intestine Meridian of Hand – Yangming, the Lung Meridian of Hand – Taiyin, the Heart Meridian of Hand – Shaoyin, and the Pericardium Meridian of Hand – Jueyin.

The 12 meridians are a virtual concept designed to study the phenomena of life, and meanwhile they correspond to the fixed areas and viscera and bowels in the human body. This is the origin of the theory of meridians and zang – fu temples in TCM. The 12 meridians in the human body connect both the organs inside and the joints outside, working together to complete the food metabolism and energy exchange of the body. Therefore, from the pathological changes in the 12 meridians and organs, we can infer abnormality of six Qi, five – zang temples and five phases of the body, and then choose the corresponding energy carrier to correct them.

五行藏象论

疾病论

On diseases

天地能量的运行是不可测的，但是有了水土的参与，能量就以风寒暑湿燥火六种气象特点表现出来。六气的本质是能量，所以六气与五行、五方、五藏、五音、五色、五味、五体、五声在能量的层面有对应关系，故内经说："东方生风，风生木，木生酸，酸生肝，肝生筋；神（能量）在天为风，在地为木，在体为筋，在藏为肝，在色为白，在音为角，在声为呼……。南方生热，热生火，火生苦，苦生心，心生血，其在天为热，在地为火，在体为脉，在藏为心，在色为赤，在音为徵，在声为笑，在味为苦，在志为喜……。中央生湿，湿生土，土生甘，甘生脾，脾生肉，其在天为湿，在地为土，在体为肉，在藏为脾，在色为黄，在音为宫，在声为歌，在味为甘，在志为思……。西方生燥，燥生金，金生辛，辛生肺，肺生皮毛，其在天为燥，在地为金，在体为皮毛，在藏为肺，在色为白，在音为商，在声为哭，在味为辛，在志为忧……。北方生寒，寒生水，水生咸，咸生肾，其在天为寒，在地为水，在体为骨，在藏为肾，在色为黑，在音为羽，在声为呻……。"

六气是天地能量的外在表现，它形成了人生存环境的空间能量场，就好像水是鱼生存的外界条件一样，适宜的水质适合鱼的生存，六气适宜有利生命活动则为正气，六气不及或过盛导致疾病则为六淫邪气。

六气是水土参与的能量形式，他们之间是可以组合的，比如风和湿的组合构成风湿，寒和燥组合成寒燥，湿和热组合成湿热。各种组合形成了复杂的能量场，这个能量场作用于人体，就会引起人体内部相应的六气变化。六气变化影响内部气血运行，气血是人体五脏六腑运行的物质载体。六气调和则气血和畅，身体健旺，六气不调则久积生病。

正常的气候变化，一年之中不同季节六气各有盛衰，并不是恒温状态，所以才有了万物的生长收藏周期。冬季当寒而寒，此寒当冬日令之气为正，若冬不寒反热，此热为冬天不当令之气，则为邪气。夏季当热反寒，此寒非夏天时令之气，为邪气。所以六气的正邪有两个含义，其一是绝对的风寒暑湿燥火盛衰，超出了大多数人的承受范围为致病邪气；其二是六气不当时令，亦为邪气。

所以适宜的寒温燥湿变化最有利于人的健康，恶劣的气候环境和失序的气候变化均影响人体内环境的稳定。中医养生讲究居住环境避风防寒，燥湿适宜，目的是为身体创造一个有益的外环境。但是天气的变化并不能保持一个标准态，如果有异常，是不是一定会导致疾病呢？答案是未必。

外界气场对身体的影响是一个方面，身体内部还有一个调节机制，就是五藏系统的自我调节。当外界六气异常可能引发内部能量场异常时，身体会通过"心肝脾肺肾"五藏之间生克耗助泄的作用，来调整气血的运行，以达到调节能量场的作用。这就是人体的适应能力，表现于外就是防病抗病能力。所以一个人的气血越充沛，五藏调节力越强，则抵御外邪的能力越强，越不容易生病。气血越差，五藏调节力越弱，则越容易生病。

同样的气候异常，有些人生病有些人保持健康，原因就在于自身五脏维持平衡的调节力。这种调节能力就是内在的正气，所谓"正气存内，邪不可干"即为此意。中国古典养生法里的导引术，不同于现代竞技体育运动，它以调整气血，强健五藏系统为目标，可以使身体元真通畅，达到无疾长寿的目的。

生病是身体内部能量运行失常导致五藏机能失调，并以身体的不适和气血水液的代谢异常表现出来，就好像四季阴阳失常以气候和自然灾害表现出来一样。人体五藏各有对应的机能，哪一藏异常则有对应症状和脉象表现，以此可以诊断内部能量运行的失常部位和原因，用改善外部能量环境和为内部提供相应属性能量的方法来纠偏。改变外部环境比如受凉之后的保暖，以暖来对治寒邪，提供能量以改变内部能量场的运行，即为药物的使用。中医里所用的药材为天地所生之动植物和矿物，每一种药材都是能量的凝聚体，通过人体的消化吸收，可以释放出其中的能量并被人体使用。

五行和六气是站在不同的角度对事物能量运动的描述。六气偏重于气化推动之力，五行偏重于相互之间的关系，五行和六气合起来就是一个完整的人体生命模型。汉代张仲景的《伤寒杂病论》就是按照这个内经理论模型，以举例说明的方式设计了一套临床药物治疗的法则。这部书成了《黄帝内经》之后，最伟大的一部医学著作。

食物带有哪种五行能量特征，就会影响到相应的五藏系统，调整能量运行和物质代谢，这就是通过食物治疗疾病的原理。口服药物属于食疗法的一种。那么药物是如何治病的呢？

四气五味

植物吸收太阳的能量，在水土参与下通过光合和呼吸作用把能量转化成物质形态，太阳的能量是植物能量的源头。而动物不能直接将太阳光转化为自身物质，需要通过直接或间接进食植物获取能量。所以区别于植物，动物有一个特殊的器官机能，就是消化系统，它能把有形的物质还原成可吸收利用的能量微粒。这个过程在水和氧气的参与下，依赖脾胃的消化吸收运化功能来完成，相当于植物通过水土来转化太阳能量。因此中医把动物的脾胃系统称做"脾土"。摄入的食物通过脾土的氤氲化合作用，化做了可以被利用的能量形式。

"化"，在古汉语里是正反、阴阳互换之意。气化为形叫"变"，形化为气叫"化"。太阳的能量变成植物形态，植物作为食物被动物吃下，被消化吸收化为动物的能量，这个生物链上传递的是太阳的能量和水土大地以及植物动物的信息。这个链条能量形式经过了两次转换，一个是大地的水土，一个是动物体的脾土。这是一个化育参赞的"变化"过程，单纯的能量在形成植物体的阶段被赋予了四气五味属性，又通过脾土将能量属性还原出来提供给动物体使用。

这个事实意味着食物中包含的四气五味属性，经过脾土运化，人体接受能量的同时，也接受了食物中包含的四气五味属性，这个属性将对人体内部的六气运行和五藏平衡产生干扰。所以四气属性过偏将对六气中的其中一气产生加强或抑制的作用，五味属性过偏，同样会影响到五藏机制，引起某一藏功能过盛或抑制。如果这种影响超出了人的调节范围，就叫做中毒。如果人体本身就有六气运转失常或五藏关系失衡，那么使用偏性的食物，却可以起到纠偏的作用，这就是中药的治疗作用。

因为正常人五藏关系和六气运行是相对平衡的，而人类又需要从饮食获得能量。所以从远古时候，人类就选择了谷物作为食物，并开始种植谷物。因为所有谷物的四气五味属性是最接近中性的，大麦、小麦、小米和水稻四气五味属性虽然有微小的差异，但是因为人体五藏系统通过生克关系有自我平衡能力，微弱的偏性不会影响到人体能量运行，所以我们祖先选择了谷物作为主要的食物来源。"四气"代表四种推动力，"五味"代表所入五藏，食物能量被脾土还原之后，温热寒凉四气化作少阳、太阳、太阴、少阴之气推动人的能量周期。酸甘苦咸辛五味各入五藏供给能量，促进五藏功能。比如单纯的酸味引起气的收敛，单纯的辛味引发气的散发，即辛散、酸收、甘缓、苦坚、咸软，任何食物从能量层面来认识，都有五行和四气的能量特征，认识了这个特征，就可以使用食物来调整人体的健康。

生活中人体受外邪内伤的影响，生长收藏化的运行并不总是稳定的，五藏平衡受内外因素的干扰也有失衡之时。不仅如此，人的生命力与动物相比，相对较弱，所以人体需要摄入酸甘苦辛咸五味和借助温热寒凉四气来调整平衡和提升生命力。而动物在一般情况下，是不需要丰富的食物种类的。所以，在人类的餐桌上除了食物之外出现了调料和各种佐料。食物和佐料气味的配和，在提供营养的同时还增加了六气动力，提升了五藏平衡能力，帮助人体建立一个动力充足的内部能量场，维持健康。

因为饮食和健康相关，所以饮食是人类重要的文明现象之一。越是历史悠久文化灿烂的民族，越拥有丰富的传统美食。中国人非常注重通过饮食来养生，是一个独特的文化现象。因为在我们的传统里，食物四气五味的能量结构与五行五藏机能对应，而五藏又包含了形气神三个层面的机能，所以食物不但影响了身体的健康，还影响了一个人的性格和精神特征。

五臭（嗅）

四气五味是食物包含的属性，每一种植物或动物带有什么样的能量属性，这种知识不是大多数人都能掌握的，这种大多属于厨师和医生的知识范畴。日常生活里我们在选择食物的时候，并不是在了解了它的属性之后才选择吃与不吃。而是通过嗅觉和味觉来决定吃与不吃，食物引起的嗅觉和味觉反应，在中医里归为五嗅范畴，肝、心、脾、肺、肾五藏对应臊、焦、香、腥、腐五嗅。人体会通过五嗅的喜好，选择食物来保证身体的需要。所以身体内部越缺少某种能量形式，你就会越喜欢吃带有这种能量特征的食物，以弥补不足，抑制有余。

幼儿脾胃娇嫩、阴阳俱虚，甘甜味属脾土，最能补充津液，甘味食物带有他们长身体最需要的能量，所以甜味是所有孩子都喜欢的味道。相对于大人来说，孩子不喜欢过于辛辣或苦咸的味道，尤其是有刺激性味道的食物，因为孩子身体的五藏系统相对平衡，没有气脉堵塞和五行偏盛，所以孩子天然不会选择特殊气味的食物。成人则不同，因为身体的隐性疾病，所以口味上有或咸或辛，或酸或辣的嗜好，这既是一种自我纠偏的行为，也是身体内部五藏失衡和气脉不通的表现。

有些家长在养育孩子的时候，根据七大营养成分的物质营养观，认为只要蛋白质脂肪等等搭配有方就可以令孩子身体健康。其实不然，因为人通过食物获取的能量是多层次的，不能仅仅理解为吃食物是建设人体有形组织的需要，正确的做法是从孩子偏好当中，认识他们的五藏需求，主动使用食物或药物来纠偏以达到平衡，其方法就是"五味生香以养五藏"。

It is impossible to predict the operation of energy contained in the universe, but the energy, with the participation of water and earth, performs with six meteorological characteristics of wind, cold, summer heat, dampness, dryness and fire. Since the nature of six meteorological phenomena, six Qi, is energy, they are correspondent from the viewpoints of energy with five phases, five directions, five – zang temples, five notes, five colors, five tastes, five body constituents, and five voices. Therefore, it says in *Yellow Emperor's Classic of Medicine*: The east engenders wind, the wind engenders wood, the wood engenders sour, the sour engenders liver, the liver engenders sinew. The spirit(energy) is the wind in the sky, and the wood on the earth, the sinew in body, the liver in the five – zang viscera, the white in the five colors, Jue in the five notes and the shout in the five voices......The south engenders summer heat, ...The heat engenders fire, the fire engenders bitter, the bitter engenders heart, the heart engenders blood. The spirit is the heat in the sky, and the fire on the earth, the pulse in the body, the heart in the five – zang temples, the red in the five colors, Zhi in the five notes and the laughter in the five voices, the bitter in the five tastes, the ecstasy in the five emotions. . . The center engenders dampness, the dampness engenders earth, the earth engenders sweet, the sweet engenders spleen, the spleen engenders flesh. The spirit is the dampness in the sky, and the earth on the earth, the flesh in the body, the spleen in the five – zang temples, the yellow in the five colors, Gong in the five notes and the singing in the five voices, the sweet in the five tastes, the anxiety in the five emotions......The west engenders dryness, the dryness engenders metal, the metal engenders spicy, the spicy engenders lung, the lung engenders skin. The spirit is the dryness in the sky, and the metal on the earth, the skin in the body, the lung in the five – zang temples, the white in the five colors, Shang in the five notes and the crying in the five voices, the spicy in the five tastes, the sadness in the five emotions. . . The north engenders cold, the cold engenders water, the water engenders salty, the salty engenders kidney. The spirit is the cold in the sky, and the water on the earth, the bone in the body, the kidney in the five – zang temples, the black in the five colors, Yu in the five notes and the groaning in the five voices.

The six meteorological phenomena or six qi are the external performance of energy in the universe, so they form the space energy field of environment where human live. Just like fish survive in the water of suitable quality. Similarly, the six meteorological phenomena which suit human activities are considered as healthy qi, while insufficient or excessive qi which results in illness are called six illed – Qi.

Since the six Qi are the energy performance with the participation of water and earth, they can combine with each other, such as, combination of wind and dampness into wind – dampness, cold and dryness into cold – dryness, dampness and summer heat into dampness – heat. The various combinations of qi form complex energy fields, and when the energy field works upon human body and it can result in corresponding changes of qi inside the body. These changes affect internal running of qi and blood which are the physical carriers of the operation of viscera. Harmonious operation of Six qi means good circulation of qi and blood and healthy body, otherwise, illness.

Normal climate change means that the six qi have a regular and dynamic change during the four seasons in a year, so there is a reasonable period of growth, flourish maturation and storage for all species on the earth. It should be cold in winter and thus the cold is considered as healthy Qi. Otherwise, If hot in winter, it is considered as illed Qi. Similarly, it should be hot in summer, if cold, it is not the right Qi in summer and considered as illed Qi. Therefore, there are two meanings for the characteristics of healthy and illed Qi in six Qi. One means that the ups and downs of six Qi, wind, cold, summer heat, dampness, dryness and fire, are absolutely beyond most people's tolerance, called pathogenic Qi causing diseases. The other one means that six Qi are not in right time in the four seasons, called pathogenic Qi.

Therefore, appropriate changes of six qi is mostly beneficial to human's health while poor environment and disorderly climate changes affect the stability of the internal environment of human body. Health preservation of TCM stresses that living environment needs to keep away wind and cold, and keep appropriate dryness and dampness in order to create a healthy external environment for human body. But the climate change can not be always normal. Does abnormal climate change certainly results in diseases? The answer is no.

中医
密码——
医之源

External qi field has an influence on body, but the internal body has a self – adjustment mechanism, i. e. , the self – adjustment of five – zang temples system. When the abnormal six qi in the external environment might lead to abnormal internal energy field of body, the body itself will adjust the running of qi and blood through the various interactions, engendering and restraining, among five – zang temples—heart temple, liver temple, spleen temple, lung temple and kidney temple, so that the energy field in the body can be adjusted. This is the adaptability of human body. It can be represented as the ability to prevent diseases. Therefore, the more abundant Qi and blood of a person and the higher adjustment ability of five – zang temples, the stronger the ability to resist pathogenic qi is and the less possibility of getting ill is. Otherwise, the poorer blood and the weaker adjustment ability of five – zang temples, the weaker the ability to resist illed qi is and the higher possibility of getting ill is.

The reason why some people get ill while some remain healthy under the same abnormal climate changes lies in the different ability of five – zang temples to keep balance. This ability is called internal healthy qi. As the Chinese saying goes, illed qi fails to impair human body when healthy qi exists inside. *Daoyin* in the classic Chinese health preservation, different from modern competitive sports, aims at adjusting qi and blood, making five – zang system strong. It is able to make the healthy Qi run in body uninterruptedly and thus achieves the goal of no illness and long life.

Getting ill arises from the abnormal operation of internal energy of human body, leading to dysfunction of five – zang temples and is represented as physical discomfort and abnormal metabolism of blood and fluid. The same goes to the big climate changes and natural calamities which are the representation of abnormal yin and yang in four seasons. Each temples has its own function, and has the corresponding symptoms and pulse conditions if abnormal. According to this, the abnormal location and the reason why it is abnormal can be diagnosed. This technique can be used to cure disease by improving external energy field and providing the corresponding needy energy for the internal body. Changing external environment works, for example, keeping warm after getting cold, using warm to treat cold illed qi. Providing the energy of medicine to change the operation of internal

疾
病
论

energy field is the use of medicine. Medicine materials used in TCM are animals, plants and minerals created by nature. Every medicine material can be seen as an energy gathering whith can release its energy to be utilized by human body through digestion and absorption.

Five phases and *six qi* are different descriptions of energy movement of different angels. *Six qi* pay attention to the driving force of energy movement while *five phases* the relationship among phases. When they are combined, an integrated human life model is constructed. *Treatise on Febrile Diseases and midcellaneous diseases* written by Zhang Zhongjing in Han dynasty, according to this Neijing theory model, designed a set of rules for clinical medicine therapy in an illustrated manner. This book has become the greatest medical work after *Yellow Emperor's Classic of Medicine*.

Food with its energy characteristic of *five phases*, influences relevant five – zang temple system when taken. It can thus adjust the energy operation and metabolism of matter. This is the principle of curing diseases by using food, i. e. food therapy. Taking oral medicine is one kind of food therapy. Then how does medicine treat disease?

Four Qi and five tastes

Plants absorb energy of the sun, and transform it into matter by photosynthesis and respiration with the participation of water and soil. The energy of the sun is the energy source of plants. While animals cannot directly transform the sunlight into matter, they need directly or indirectly feed on plants to get energy. What sets animals apart from plants is that animals have a special organ system, the digestive system, which can transform tangible food into energy microparticles to be used by the body. This process is completed by the digestion, assimilation and transformation functions of the spleen and stomach system with the participation of water and oxygen, which is similar to plants transforming the energy of the sun *via* water and soil. That's why the traditional Chinese medicine calls the spleen – stomach system "spleen – earth". spleen – earth is used to transform food to the energy which can be used by the body. "Hua" in ancient Chinese words means the process of interconverstion between pros and cons or Yin and Yang.

The process of Qi converted into tangible matter is called"change"(bian) , and that of the tangible matter converted into Qi is called"transform"(hua) . The energy of the sun converts into plants, and plants are eaten by animals, which are absorbed and changed into animal's energy. This food chain passes the information about the energy of the sun and information of water, earth, vegetation and animals. The energy of food chain is transformed twice, one by water and soil, the other by the spleen – earth of animals. This is a breeding process of change, during which pure energy changes into plants, and is endowed with the attributes of four Qi and five tastes, then these attributes are restored by spleen – earth for the body to use.

The fact means that after the assimilation of spleen – earth, the attributes of the four Qi and the five tastes that food has, are accepted by the body when it gets the energy. And the attributes will interfere with the six – qi operation of body and the balance among five – zang temples. Therefore, if the attributes of the four Qi are lopsided, they will reinforce or restrain one of the six – qi, and if the attributes of the five tastes are lopsided, they will also exert an effect on the operation mechanism of five – zang temples, finally making one of the five – zang temples too strong or too weak. If the effect is beyond man's regulation, it will cause food poisoning. If the balance of the six – qi and five – zang temples has already been broken, then using lopsided food can correct the imbalance, which is the treatment principle of traditional Chinese medicine.

As the five – zang temples, relations and six – qi operation are relatively balanced for normal people, and people need to eat for energy. Since primitive times, man has chosen grains as their food, and begun to grow grains. That's because four qi and five tastes of grains are the most balanced. Grains such as barley, wheat, millet, rice vary slightly in nature, and these slight deviations cannot affect the operation of energy in the body because the five – zang temples system has the ability to keep a balance through engendering and restraining function. That's why our ancestors chose grains as the main food. Four Qi represent four kinds of impetus, five tastes represent the corresponding five – zang temples. After the energy of food is restored by spleen – earth, the four qi of warm, hot, cold and

疾
病
论

cool change into the qi of *shao – yang, tai – yang, tai – yin, shao – yin* to promote the progression of man's energy circulation. The five tastes are sour, sweet, bitter, salty, spicy, invading the five – zang temples, and supplying energy for them and making sure that they function well. For example, pure sour causes Qi to astringe, and pure spicy causes Qi to dissipate, that is, spicy causes dissipation, sour causes astringency, sweet causes relaxation, bitter causes hardness, salty causes softness. Any food has the attribute of the five phases and the four Qi from the viewpoint of energy. The knowledge of these attributes, makes it possible to use food to promote health.

In daily life, as the human body is affected by external pathogen andinternal damage, the transformation functions among"growth, flourish maturation and storage"are not stable, the balance of five – zang temples can be disturbed by inside and outside factors. Besides, human's vitality is not as good as other animals. Therefore, people need to take in the five tastes of sour, sweet, bitter, salty and spicy, and four – qi of warm, hot, cold and cool to keep balance and promote vitality, while other animals generally do not need a variety of food. Accordingly, there are not only food but also flavors and condiments on people's dining table. Food mixed with condiments and flavors provides nutrition and six – qi impetus, promotes the balance ability of five – zang temples, and assists the body to build a strong internal energy field to keep healthy.

As closely related to health, diet is one of the most important civilized phenomena in human's history. The longer the history and the more prosperous the culture a nation has, the more abundant traditional food there is. Chinese people pay much attention to diet to stay healthy, which is a unique cultural phenomenon. As in our tradition, the energy structure of food, four – qi and five – taste, correspond to the five phases and five – zang temples, and the five – zang temples contain three – level functions of figure, qi and spirit. That's why food not only determines physical health, but also affects people's characters and spirit.

Five smells

Four Qi and five tastes are the attributes of food, what kind of energy attribute every plant or animal carries is not known to most people, for this kind of expertise is the specialty of a cook or a doctor. When we choose food in daily life, we do not need to know all these attributes to decide whether to eat or not, instead we decide by the smell and taste. The response evoked by the smell and taste of the food, can be categorized into five smells. The five – zang temples, the liver, heart, spleen, lungs and kidneys temple, correspond to the five smells, which are urine, burnt, aroma, fishy and rotten, respectively. People choose food by their preference for the five smells to meet the body's requirement. Accordingly, the scarcer energy there is in the body, the more likely one likes to eat the food with this energy attribute to make up for the shortage.

Baby's spleen – stomach is tender and weak in both *yin* and *yang*. Sweet corresponds to spleen – earth, and can supplement fluid and humor. Sweet food can bring energy which is the most indispensable to their growth. That's why sweet is children's favorite flavor. Compared with adults, children dislike food that is too spicy or salty, especially pungent food. Because children's five – zang system is relatively balanced, the Qi channel is neither blocked nor are the five phases lopsided, they do not choose food with special flavors. While for adults, they usually have hidden diseases, so they prefer food that is salty or spicy, sour or hot. That's a activity of self – correction, a sign of the imbalance of their five – zang temples or the qi channels being blocked.

Some parents think that by the nutriology theory of seven nutrients, as long as protein and fat and other nutrients can be arranged in proper proportions, then it can make children grow up healthily. That's not the case. Because the energies human gets from food are multi – layered, it is more than eating to meet the need of building the physical body. The right way is to find their five zang's requirements from their dietary preferences, then to use relative food or medicine to rectify the deviation and strike a balance. The solution summarized here is "making use of five smells to nourish the five – zang temples".

四气五味与中医营养观

Four Qi, five tastes and TCM nutriology

食物是能量的聚集态，身体通过摄取食物获得能量。能量有五种基本形式，起到推动身体生长收脏和物质建设的功能。所以食物的营养就分为两种，一种是推动之力，称之为卫气，与"温热寒凉"四气相关；一种是建设有形组织器官的功能称为营气，与"酸甘苦辛咸"五味相关。

现代流行的营养观认为人体的营养素由蛋白质、脂质、碳水化合物、维生素、矿物质、水和纤维素七类成分构成。谷物、肉类、蔬菜和水果是最主要的食物来源。如果以这种营养学的观点来看食物，那么苹果和菠萝，生姜和大葱在营养成分上是没有多少区别的。如果这个观点成立，那就意味着不论什么种类的食物，只要营养素全面对身体产生的效果都是一样的。

实际情况并非如此，植物会因其品种、产地、生长季节和储存方式的不同，集聚不同的能量和信息。同样是大米，生长在东北五常的大米和生长在湖北的转基因大米，从形状、口感和营养价值上差异巨大。新疆的羊肉和东海的带鱼也是气味完全不同的食物，但是它们却可能具有相同的蛋白质和脂肪比例。

所以食物营养不仅仅是七大基本元素这种有形部分，食物还有四气五味属性，五味对应五行和五藏。大多数人会有这么一种体会，有时候会特别馋某样食物有食之而后快的冲动，这就是身体通过口味选择调节五脏平衡的机制在发挥作用。中医可以通过一个人的口味来了解五行盛衰，然后选择相应的食物或药材给予纠偏以维持五藏平衡，这种方法用于日常保健叫做食疗，用于治病叫做药疗。

相同的两块羊肉，用清水煮熟和加作料煮熟，味道是不同的，后者滋味醇厚浓香，叫滋补羊肉汤，前者清汤寡水，估计没人喜欢吃。这是因为加了食盐、茴香、八角、大料、肉桂的羊肉经过水火氤氲和化，形成了一种新的物质状态。就好像天地气交产生的气候之变，其能量状态既不同于之前的天道能量，也不同于地道能量。加佐料熬制好的羊肉汤醇厚香浓，是因为各种食材化和之后形成了第三种能量场。因为"香"入脾，脾主运化，所以熬制后羊肉的能量更容易被充分吸收。在熬制的时候加入了各种佐料，所以四气五味调和滋养五脏的同时，还提升了五脏的机能。因此，羊肉汤本身就形成了一个五行俱全、气味协调的能量场，对身体起到的营养作用不同于单纯的羊肉。

辛、酸、甘、苦、咸五味，各有温热寒凉和生长收藏化的功能，酸入肝，辛入肺，苦入心，咸入肾，甘入脾。辛散、酸收、甘缓、苦坚、咸软，故四气五味属性可用于调整身体内部的能量场，既能养生保健又能遣方治病。

以中医营养学的观点来看，四气五味不全，或者调配不当滋味不佳，都属于营养失当。很多人误以为清淡就是健康饮食，其实对大部分人来说，这造成了气味的缺乏，反而不利于身体健康。以中医的观点来看，健康的饮食观点是"量出为入，气味调和，五味俱全，色好味美"，懂得了食物四气五味的搭配，也就懂得了中药的搭配。

四气五味的形成与道地药材论

来自宇宙空间的能量是无差别的，这个能量被大地吸收然后再散射出去，就带有了该地的能量属性。天地能量的交汇是在特定区域内地脉水土的参与下完成的，局部的气候条件形成的小环境能量场，就有能量特性上的差异。

同一种植物有其基本的能量属性，但是生长在不同的小环境里，因为依赖于小环境的能量场交换，故在基本属性的基础上，在基因赋予的能量特征之外又添加了生长区域内的能量信息特点。所以同一颗种子，在不同的地区，长成之后其性质是有差异的，这种差异既表现在外部物理性状的不同，也表现在内部能量信息的差异。

总有一些地区的能量场对某种植物的生长特别适宜，而且可以最大限度的增加这种植物的能量属性。与他处移栽者相比，所贮存的能量信息最纯正充沛，气味最足，比如西湖的龙井茶、阳澄湖的大闸蟹、宁夏的枸杞、新会的陈皮。这就叫做当地的土特产，如果这种植物用来做药材，就叫做"道地药材"。

道地药材是指生长在特定自然条件和生态环境下的药材，此种药材在这个区域内生长能量特性充足，改变人体能量场最有效。

Food is the aggregation state of energy, and the body gets energy by eating food. There are five basic forms of energy, which promote the "growth, flourish maturation and storage" and rebuilding of cells in the body. There are two kinds of nutrients in food. One is the driving force, called defensive Qi, which is related to the four qi of warm, hot, cold and cool. The other is the function of rebuilding organs, called nutrient Qi, which is related to the five tastes of sour, sweet, bitter, salty and spicy.

In modern times the most popular nutrition notion is that there are seven nutrients needed by the body which are protein, fat, carbohydrate, vitamin, minerals, water and fiber. Grains, meat, vegetables and fruit are the main source of food. If observed from the perspective of nutriology, there is no much difference in nutrients between the ginger and shallot, apple and pineapple. If the nutriology notion is valid, that means whatever food it is, as long as the nutrients are comprehensive, the effects on the body are the same.

That is not the case. Plants may contain different energy and information because of different species, growing areas and seasons as well as storage. For example, Rice grown in Wuchang, Northeast China and the genetically modified rice grown in Hubei are different in shape, taste and nutritive value. Mutton produced in Xinjiang and hairtail grown in the East China Sea are different kinds of food with different flavors, but they maybe have the same protein and fat proportion.

Accordingly, the nutrition of food is more than the visible part of the seven nutrients, there are the attributes of the four Qi and the five tastes. The five tastes correspond to the five phases and five – zang temples. Many people have the experience of hungering for some kind of food at times, that's the body's mechanism — coordinating the five – zang balance by choice of taste—is working. A TCM doctor can know the surplus and deficiency of the five phases by one's preference for taste, and then choose the corresponding food or medicine to modify and balance the five – zang temples. The method used to keep fit in daily life is called dietary therapy, to treat an illness is called medical therapy.

The same two pieces of mutton taste differently if one is cooked with just water and the other cooked with condiment. The latter tastes delicious and is nourishing while the former is tasteless and it is likely that no one likes it. That's because when the mutton cooked with condiments such as salt, fennel seeds, star anise, cinnamon and so on, it changes into a new state. Just as when the sky qi and the earth qi meet, the weather changes. The energy generated not only differs from the energy of sky, but also differs from the energy of the earth. The mutton cooked with condiments tastes aromatic because the fusion of condiments and mutton forms a new energy field. As aroma invades the spleen, which is in charge of transportation and transformation, then the energy of the later mutton is easier to be fully assimilated. Because of the added condiments when cooking, the four qi and the five tastes generated not only nourish the five – zang temples, but also promote the five – zang's functions. Therefore, the mutton soup becomes an energy field which is complete in the five phases and has the harmonized qi and taste, its nutrition is more than the former one with only mutton.

The five tastes of sour, sweet, bitter, salty and spicy, have the attributes of warm, hot, cold, and cool and the functions of growth, flourish maturation, storage and transformation. Sour invades the liver temple, similarly, spicy invades the lungs temple, bitter invades the heart temple, salty invades the kidney temple, and sweet invades the spleen temple. As pure sour causes astringency, pure spicy causes dissipation, sweet causes relaxation, bitter causes hardness, and salty causes softness, so the attributes of four qi and five tastes can be used to adjust the energy field of the body, to make people healthier and cure the sickness.

From the viewpoint of TCM nutriology, lack of four qi or five tastes, or improper arrangement leading to bad taste, is improper diet. Many people have the misconception that a light diet means a healthy diet, but for most people, that results in the lack of flavors, doing no good to health. From the viewpoint of Chinese Traditional medicine, the principle of healthy diet is "to strike a balance between the input and output, keep taste and qi in harmony, the five tastes being all complete, be delightful to see and smell. " Knowing how to collocate the four qi and five tastes of food, means knowing how to collocate Chinese medicine.

四气五味与中医营养观

Formation of four qi and five tastes and theory of genuine medicinal herbs

The energy from cosmic space is indiscriminate, and it is absorbed and dissipated by the earth, then it has the energy attribute of the earth. Since the energy of the sky and the energy of the earth merge together with the participation of water and soil of the given area, the climates of different locations form different microervironments, which have different attributes of energy.

Plants of the same species have the same basic attribute, but as they grow in different smallenvironments, and depend on the exchange of energy field in the smallenvironments, besides the genetic energy attribute they have the characteristics of the energy and information of the growing area. Therefore, the same seed may have different attributes when it grows in different places, both different in external physical shapes and intemal energy and information.

There are always some places which are very suitable for one kind of plant, and can maximize the energy attribute of the plant. Compared with plants in other places, the plant there has the purest energy information and the strongest smell, such as the Longjing tea grown around the West Lake area, the hairycrab in Yangcheng Lake, wolfberry in Ningxia, the tangerine peel(chenpi) in Xinhui. This is called local specialty, if the plant is used for medicine, it is called genuine medicinal herb.

Genuine medicinal herbs are medical herbs grown in specific natural conditions and environment, which have the maximum energy, and are most effective in changing the body's energy field.

陈皮的故事

The story of Chenpi
(tangerine peel)

（上）

儿时记忆中陈皮指放久的橘子皮，小时候吃橘子的时候会把橘子皮剥来晾晒在窗台上。因为大点的孩子总是以认真的表情告诉我，橘子皮晾干之后就变成了一味中药，可以治病，所以我会自觉的把橘子皮积攒起来。虽然不知道哪一天会用上，但都会很认真的去做这件事。（童年时很多知识，就是这样接受下来的。）

小时候不但晾晒橘皮还晾晒鸡内金，就是鸡的胃壁黏膜，因为鸡内金可以治疗消化不良。去住农村的小伙伴家里玩，总能发现他们从地头田边摘来的花花草草晾晒在院子里。他们会指着这些东西说出它们的名字，然后告诉我它们各自能治疗什么病。印象最深的是去一个新认识的朋友家里，他趁家里大人不在，带我看养在大竹篮子里的毒蝎子。这些药材都是可以卖钱补贴家用的，而且大部分的劳动都是孩子们在做，想一想七八岁时的种种贪玩之举，无意中竟然埋下了关于中医的回忆。

20 世纪 70 年代做了父母的那一拨人，经历过社教和破四旧，大多数人已经不相信中医的土方验方能治病了。思想改造彻底点的青年父母，甚至会以相信中医治病为耻，认为是迷信、不科学的。我自己就生活在这样的城市里，所以没有体验更丰富的传统生活方式，也因此成了一件憾事。所有的天材地宝都是从土地上长出来的，知识就是如此，只有接地气多层次的生活体验，才会养育出智慧，学校的教育在这个里面只起一部分的作用。

朋友带来了道地药材

前些天一位朋友到访，带来了他花费半年时间，走遍全国各地淘来的宝贝。他说这些新宝贝带给他的快乐远胜过去收藏的古董和字画，要与我分享。他所说的宝贝其实是几种很常见的植物类药材，只是品质不同，就好像正宗的西湖龙井和普通茶叶的差异一样。所带之物中，有长得近似血管的广西桂枝，不但管径、管壁、管腔与人体血管极似，而且气味特足。闻一鼻子后脑勺风府穴微微发胀，热血欲腾，立马有从座位上站起来甩甩胳膊活动一下的冲动，这个形状和气味与桂枝温通血脉的作用非常吻合。

有一味形状如同结肠一样的野生鸡矢藤，藤条横断面的形状酷似大肠皱襞。结肠的黏膜层和肌肉层的形状在这个藤断面有惟妙惟肖的体现，而且管径也与结肠类似，散发出来的气味直入下腹，让人产生欲排便的感觉。气味这么足，对人的气血运行影响这么大，说明朋友找来的是道地药材。他之所以这么开心，是因为中药的使用量太大，道地药材的产量有限，所以大多数药材都非原产地所出。即便在原产地，因为要追求产量，农药化肥大量使用，也会使药物质量下降。而且采收时间的不严格和以及保存上的问题，真正高质量的道地药材其实很少，野生的就更为难得，能得到当然令其欢喜不已。

道地药材为什么效果不同？举个例子就容易理解，同样的葡萄，新疆吐鲁番种植的就会格外甜。现在的中医大夫有一个缺陷，对药性的了解来源于书本而不是实践，对药材只知其名不知其形味，所以对药物的作用都很难有切身的认识。这也造成了治病开方不是利用药材遣兵布阵，而是医者对描写药材功效的文字进行排列组合。这种间接的知识体验，就好像厨师没有体验过盐的咸味，却要根据食者的口味调味一样。大家能想象一个没有品尝过调料的厨师，根据对调料的文字描述，就能做出一桌好菜的师傅吗？而现在医学院培养出的医生基本上属于这种厨师。所以我曾建议爱好中医的这位朋友，每味药都最好能自己体验。结果他慢慢发现药房里的药材太不靠谱，很难达到古书里记载的那种药效。原因不是古书错了，而是药材不地道，所以这位用心的朋友就开始了他人生中的寻找道地药材之旅。这个过程给他带来了一次又一次的惊喜，这几包简单的药材里，一定藏着他不一般的故事和快乐。所以，那天下午基本上是他在讲述寻找和辨别药材的经历。

新会陈皮

朋友拿出一袋当年的新会陈皮，这个陈皮颜色就好像吃过不久的柑子皮，颜色绿中带黄。陈皮的"陈"指的是陈旧的意思，顾名思义，放置的时间越久，药性越好。所以好的陈皮颜色比较深，朋友拿出来的这个陈皮显然不怎么陈，没有乌沉沉的那种品相，就好像吃过之后随手丢弃的橘柑皮，且听他如何讲述。他说这个陈皮是从当地药农家里收购的，开始只是为了去广州新会买点上好陈皮，药农见他对药材特别认真，就给他说了实话。告诉他现在卖的任何年份的陈皮，其实都是通过技术手段做旧出来的，外观跟陈茶似的，其实都不是陈年老货。实际上能买到当地的陈皮就很不错了，因为销量大，当地很多陈皮是外地运来的柑皮上色加工而成，因为当地陈皮没有那么大的产量。后来带朋友去他自己家里，教他如何鉴别陈皮，并且说真的想要得

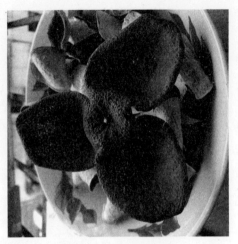

图 22 - 2　"新会陈皮"

到陈年陈皮，只能自己存放，现在每年的陈皮一出来就卖完啦，根本没有多余的库存。听他这么一说，我也长了知识。朋友带来的陈皮是当年新货，故而颜色黄绿，细观陈皮表面满布细孔，对光可看到皮层有一层油滴，近毛孔处更明显，如同放大镜下人的皮肤。挨近鼻孔深吸一口气，感觉气味先沉降入腹，后味中有清香之气，这股清香上行至咽喉处，气味层次丰富，前味和后味的气味以及最后在身体上的停留点均不相同，符合古书所载味厚气薄的特征。

聊天过程中，摘了半瓣陈皮当功夫茶泡。过去说药方吃对了，下咽就有作用。我是痰湿体质，所以平时嗓音比较低沉。喝了两杯之后，忽然感到嗓子发干，我知道这是药起作用了。清了一下嗓子，同样的语音，突然发觉声音比喝茶前变亮了，而且周围人也觉察到了这个变化，相视一笑，喜不自胜，说明这个药材是真的。

嗓子发干是因为积聚在喉间的痰湿被清除，声音自然就会变得敞亮。这是陈皮起到了理气消痰、清咽利喉的作用。而且只有上升到咽喉的气味尚存，才会有此作用。人体津液在热茶的带动下上行，到第四杯的时候，嗓子的里面由干涩变为清爽，身体也出现微微的轻快之感。这是陈皮后味在发挥作用。古人说陈皮味厚气薄，属阴中之阳能上达咽喉。如果陈皮被烤箱烤过，外形虽然没有变化，但烤箱的燥性破坏了陈皮的清香上行之气，所以清咽利喉，理气消痰的作用就减弱了。而且烤箱烤过之后，陈皮

上面的一层油脂被耗干，没有这个东西，陈皮大部分药性会由此丧失，那就成了徒有其形的陈皮，完全不是古书里所载的药材陈皮了。

天地之间，不管是人还是物，缺了那口气，就不是那个东西啦。故曰"人不可夺志，药不可夺气，三军不可夺帅"。获得知识的途径，古人说"生而知之者上，学而知之者次之"，那么怎么才能知道陈皮的作用呢？古人有一种高明的学习方法叫取象比类。

陈皮第一个明显的特征是陈皮为水果之皮，那么它和万物之中一切表皮都有同频共振的效果，所以药性发挥的部位首先与表皮有关。在人体，覆盖于身体表面的皮肤还有覆盖于内脏表面的表皮以及脏腑内壁的黏膜，都属于表皮的范畴。我们把陈皮拿在手上细看是不是特别像人的皮肤？不但有纹路相似的表面，还有均匀分布的毛孔，而且最外层还覆盖有一层薄薄的油脂。晾干之后透光而看特别像动物的皮革，而在放大镜下，又非常类似于人体皮肤的结构。这是陈皮正面给我们的印象。

不仅如此，再看陈皮的内面，简直就是一个完美的人体皮下组织标本：白色的内皮和网状结构相当于真皮组织和皮下黏膜，即中医里面所说的腠理。陈皮就是表皮和腠理的结合体。这给了我们一个很大的提示，就是陈皮和皮肤在信息层面是有同频之处的，所以陈皮对皮肤一定有影响。那么究竟是什么样的影响，就由陈皮的四气五味特性决定。作用于皮肤这个位置，是陈皮的药理特征，而且可能是基础作用，其他的一切效用，都是建立在这个作用之上的效果，事实是不是如此呢？

橘络

吃柑橘的时候，橘皮和橘瓣之间有一层丝丝拉拉的橘络，这个橘络和橘皮一样也是一味中药。白色的橘络分布于橘瓣和橘皮之间，互相连通没有间断。其颜色和形状颇似连接人体脏腑和体腔之间的筋膜。这层筋膜在人体叫做三焦筋膜，是元气通行于五脏六腑的通道。橘络晒干之后作用于三焦筋膜，而陈皮作用位置偏向于表皮层，两者性味相似而作用点不同。那么这个表皮仅仅是指人体表面的皮肤吗？当然不是，人体每个脏腑表面都覆盖有一层表皮，生物学上称之为浆膜。这层表皮把内脏和体腔内的环境隔开，五脏六腑通过这层表皮与内环境进行能量和信息的交换。陈皮同样可以作用于这些脏腑的表皮细胞。除过浆膜这层表皮之外，呼吸道和胃肠道，甚至膀胱这些空腔脏器的内表面，都有一层单层表皮细胞覆盖，这层细胞主导人体的吸收分泌作用，也属于内外交换的门户。

生命存活的基础是内外环境的物质交换，在细胞层面此规律也可以体现为组织细胞的内外交换。这一切都是通过表皮这个门户来进行的。那么一旦有代谢废物堆积，影响到了新陈代谢，这个堆积最容易发生在哪里？当然是交换最频繁的门户区。陈皮以其苦而辛温的气味特点，起到清泻附着在脏腑表面垃圾的作用，从而清洁了人体内外物质和能量交换通路。这种作用于表皮的功能覆盖了生物学上的单层扁平上皮和复层扁平上皮，而这两种细胞覆盖了人体所有的脏腑。陈皮能清理堆积在各脏腑门户里的垃圾，这就是在中医里陈皮治疗范围特别广泛的原因。

古人总结陈皮的作用，认为其可以"理气消痰，治大便闭涩，治上气咳嗽"，这是作用于肺与大肠的表皮起到的作用；"定呕哕嘈杂，开胃和中"这是作用于胃肠道上皮细胞起到的作用。古人认为陈皮能除膀胱留热及停水，这个作用今天很难理解，但仔细分析，膀胱内外也是一层黏膜和浆膜层上皮包裹，如果这一层的门户受堵，则内外交换不畅而生寒热，影响水道通利。用中医"取象比类"的思考方法，陈皮的这一作用就容易理解了。

最经典的《神农本草经》言陈皮能利水谷，水谷为后天之气行走于三焦筋膜，利水谷其实就是通利三焦之气，这正好对应于陈皮内面以及橘络之特征。如果记不住那么多的功效，你就把陈皮想象成在官宦门前手执扫帚清理门户的那个仆人，陈皮的作用就全记住了。金元时期有个叫张元素的医家认为"陈皮能泻、能散、能和、能温、能补，化痰治嗽，顺气理中，调脾快膈，其功在诸药之上"。明代李时珍赞"陈皮味苦，能泻能燥，味辛能散，善治百病"，原因在于它理气燥湿的功效。陈皮打扫垃圾是有条件的，门户有郁堵才发挥作用，门户没有郁堵却用之，不但无效，反而消耗气血。

善用陈皮

在中医兴趣聊天群里，发生过这样的事，因为了解到陈皮的作用，感觉对身体特别好，积极的妈妈马上给孩子做了陈皮米粥喝，这样有益吗？陈皮的使用是有条件的，就是有垃圾堆积才可以使用。孩子身体是比较通畅的，没有那么多的油腻秽物，所以孩子就排斥陈皮的味道。不仅陈皮，很多对成人来说很喜欢的味道，孩子都不能接受，比如辣椒、大蒜、芫荽、小茴香和胡椒等等，其原因就在于体质的差异。如果孩子喜欢一些特殊的口味，就代表身体内部可能有相应的问题。

陈皮在食品行业又叫青红丝，小时候吃的月饼里面都加有青红丝。因为月饼比较油腻，加了青红丝，就能及时清理门户，保持交换通畅，不容易被油腻堵住上皮组织。所以从效果上看就是加了青红丝之后便于消化，不会积食。除此之外煮肉、做八宝甜米饭这种高能量食品时，加青红丝可以促进吸收。如果一个人偶尔吃得太多，腹胀气喘，这时候用陈皮泡水去去痰气，更利于气脉流通。大家知道为什么胖人易短寿吗？就是因为垃圾堆积阻碍了三焦气脉的运行。陈皮能清理垃圾行气，从这个角度说，陈皮有保持健康长寿的作用。后世医家以"消滞气"来定义陈皮的作用，如果以此来理解，则无法善用陈皮，宋代医家张元素言其具有能泻、能散等"五能作用"，在对陈皮这味药的解释上，远胜于诸多医家。先生就是历史上创造中药归经理论的张洁古前辈。

新会陈皮的历史

有名的广州新会陈皮其实不是橘皮而是柑皮。新会陈皮的出名，源于黄姓家族的一个女人米氏。距今七百年前南宋理宗年间，杨太后患乳疾。米氏作为贵族女子此时正好诏侍于杨太后，用新会家中自制的陈皮给太后服用而起效，太后病愈之后，封米氏为"邦显一品夫人"。米氏诏侍期满回家之后教授族人广种柑树，制作陈皮作为药用。从此新会陈皮名扬天下，中药谱里新增一味被称为"广陈皮"的中药，其药性与之前的橘皮类似而力道更强。慢慢的广陈皮就代替了橘皮，此后数百年直到民国，在新会银洲湖和潭江、西江下游制作贩卖广陈皮的黄氏子弟历代不绝。高峰时十户有七八户从事此业，开创了广陈皮走遍海内外，领衔天下七百年的历史。

（下）

陈皮表面附着有一层油泡，行家认为这层油泡越丰厚，陈皮的质量越好。新会陈皮之所以出名，也与其油脂含量比其他地区高有关，水谷之气为人体后天之气，合于真气而充身周内外，若水谷之气受阻沉积于气道，则造成痰气壅胀。清除堆积的油腻之物，需要两个条件：一是溶解，二是推动。前面在《四气五味》篇里我们讲过，辛能散，苦能坚。推动来自于陈皮的苦辛之气，溶解则源于陈皮本身所含的油泡。

这有点像中学化学里学到的极性溶液溶解极性分子，非极性溶液溶解非极性分子的道理：含油泡充足的陈皮能更好的分解上皮层附着的油腻之物，所以消痰的作用更好。如果没有油泡，陈皮苦辛之味就成了纯推动的行气作用，就好像没有洗洁精而直接用清水冲刷油碗，不能化掉痰浊而只能散气。有人提倡用新会陈皮泡水来预防雾霾引起的尘肺，陈皮化痰的原理是通过散、泻、温、清理堆积于门户的垃圾。陈皮能治胃肠垃圾导致的呕哕嘈杂，时吐清水以及因为脾湿运化不足导致的脾肺痰湿。如此使用陈皮是最适当的。但是雾霾中 PM2.5 范围内的微尘颗粒由外而来，这种颗粒堆积在肺泡以及肺泡与肺泡的中间组织之间，非水谷之气，所以喝陈皮水不能达到清理雾霾中微尘颗粒的作用。

大家可能会有一个疑问，同样是陈皮，为什么时间越久越值钱呢？存放日久的陈皮物性有什么变化吗？是的，在不同的时空环境下，任何生命性质都会发生变化，只是这种变化不是五官能明显感受得到而已。刚从树上摘下来的新鲜水果，有酸涩之味，并不好吃。放置一段时间后，味道就会有变化，这是因为果实离开枝头后，它的生命支行其实并没有停止。陈皮在储藏阶段，仍然在发生着性质的变化。任何一个生命体，时时刻刻都在与周围的时空环境进行着信息和能量的交换。霜降之后的柿子味道会变得甘甜，立春之后就不好吃了，这是外界气场的改变对柿子造成的影响。泡菜缸半截埋到土里腌出来的味道比单元楼房里腌制的味道好，这是地气对泡菜的影响。储存陈皮和储存茶叶一样，采摘之后在四季轮换的岁月里，会继续发生变化。种植陈皮的药农说，2016 年冬天天气不冷，所以

2016 年的新陈皮就是黄绿色。如果天气很冷，陈皮就是变成了红色，而红色陈皮味道更好。

初晒的陈皮性温和醇绵之气不足，久置陈皮生涩之味失而醇厚之味生。味厚油气增则化痰清利温补之性增强，因为前面唱的陈皮年份短，所以加了陈皮熟潽一起泡，期望达到老陈皮的效果。普洱与陈皮同泡，其实就蕴含了药物炮制之理。包括用柑皮制作的青红丝，都属于中药炮制范畴。

无独有偶，喝过陈皮汤那天下午，一位家在湖北荆州的妈妈从 QQ 上发来一组照片和文字消息，因为孩子过年积食上火，按照偏方，吃了三颗当地的臭皮柑子而速好，故留言与我，转录于此：

1. "荆州这种酸柑子，当地人说清火效果好，二哥知道这种水果不？又苦又酸。"

2. "百度说性味辛，苦，温，去寒化痰，但当地人都说去火的，嘴巴打泡，干燥裂口，嗓子不舒服，连吃三个酸柑子就好了，胜过任何良药，这和度娘说的去寒有出入，难道这个水果寒热通吃？"

3. "人可以寒热同时存在，那有既清热又祛寒，同时双功效的植物么？"

4. "百度找到学名了：臭皮柑和柚子有点相似，要分清柚子和臭皮柑很简单，臭皮柑比柚子小一点，表皮比橘子更粗糙一点。臭皮柑，吃起来又苦又酸，可是它的药性却非常好，很多人把它拿回家，加蜂蜜腌制，做成蜂蜜臭皮柑，对治疗咳嗽、化痰清淤很有效。明朝李时珍《本草纲目》中，记载："臭皮柑佳品，利气、化痰、止咳功倍于它药……其功愈陈愈良。"清朝《本草纲目拾遗》记载："臭皮柑治痰症，消油腻、消食、醒酒、宽中、解蟹毒。"

这位妈妈也是中医爱好者，所以给孩子连吃三个臭皮柑后积食上火之症竟然好了，惊喜之余与我有了如上交流。我告诉她这次回老家认识了一味好药，臭皮柑应该和新会制作陈皮的大红柑同属于药用之材。我建议她多收集一些带回深圳，最好是用蜂蜜腌制一些。对容易积食的孩子，还有痰湿较重的大人可以清理食积和痰壅。

臭皮柑清火是清的胃肠道食积肉积形成的实火，其辛苦散泻的作用，清理了肠道内的壅堵之物，胃肠道之火降下去，所以孩子的上火症状就好啦。并不是臭柑子属温性便不能去火，这里用的治疗方法不是以寒治热，

陈皮的故事

而是清理垃圾而达到胃肠调和的目的。假如肠道没有垃圾，吃了臭皮柑，正常的津液被排出体外，津液少加上臭皮柑的温性，吃多了反倒容易上火，尤其是对于津液虚的小孩子，更是如此。所以中医讲究对症下药，中病即止。

这位妈妈遇到的医学问题说明万物没有绝对的好坏，用的对就有益，用的不对则有害。

陈皮的使用

广东化州产的橘红也属于陈皮之中的名品，俗称"化橘红"，以片薄大，色橙红，质油润，橘络多者为佳。这是为什么呢？

道理和新会陈皮是一样的，只是毛居多，其形状更接近皮肤。肺主皮毛，所以化橘红在治疗肺痰时更甚其他种类的陈皮。

为什么陈皮均以油脂多而为上品呢？人体痰浊堆积之物多有油脂，万物无同频则无相吸，陈皮有了油脂，发挥清理人体痰浊垃圾时就有了向导。

陈皮最显著的作用就是理气消痰。有一个有名的除痰方剂叫二陈汤，非常适用于现代人多吃少动造成的痰湿体质，以及由痰湿体质形成的各种现代疾病，比如高血脂，高血糖，以及关节疾病。

该方组成为半夏、陈皮、茯苓和炙甘草，四味药磨成粉，每次取10克，加生姜数片，乌梅一枚，水煎温服，只饮水不喝药渣。此方能燥湿化痰，理气和中，是治疗寒湿化痰的基本方。

湿痰堆积在胃肠则胃失和降，恶心呕吐；堆积于胸膈之间则气机不畅，痞闷不舒；堆积于肺则咳嗽痰多，肺失宣降，喘而大便不畅；阻三焦脉气运行，痰湿水气不行，则头目眩晕；痰浊阻于心脉，则心悸，面恍白，心虚多疑，因为心其华在面；阻于脾土肌肉，则肢体困重；

陈皮苦降辛散之性还能将痰湿排出体外；茯苓除水湿，此方通过清除痰饮水湿病理物质而起效；半夏性燥故能燥湿化痰；陈皮苦辛故能行痰化痰。此方要求半夏、橘红皆取陈久者用，故方名"二陈"汤。半夏加陈皮是祛痰方剂中理气化痰的常用组合。

"二陈汤"中，生姜色黄质厚味辛，入于胃行于肺，肺胃动而水谷之气行，煎加生姜，起协助陈皮半夏排痰之功。若有痰湿阻胃，生姜是必用之物。《金匮要略》中，陈皮生姜组合治胃气上逆，是辛温行气的典型方剂，而生姜半夏汤用生姜汁入药，增加此方生姜辛开之功；用少许乌梅，防止辛燥伤津导致上火之虞。

二陈汤的变化使用：

治湿痰，可加苍术、厚朴以增燥湿化痰之力；

治热痰，可加胆星、瓜蒌以清热化痰；

治寒痰，可加干姜、细辛以温化寒痰；

治风痰眩晕，可加天麻、僵蚕以化痰熄风；

治食痰，可加莱菔子、麦芽以消食化痰；

治郁痰，可加香附、青皮、郁金以解郁化痰；

治痰流经络之瘰疬、痰核，可加海藻、昆布、牡蛎以软坚化痰。

陈皮的故事至此结束。

(First part)

According to my memory in childhood, *chenpi* referred to the peel of the tangerine that was long stored. In my childhood, when I ate the tangerine, I would peel it first, and then place the peel on the windowsill to dry it. Older children always told me with a serious look that the tangerine peel would become a herbal medicine after being dried and aired, and could cure diseases, so I would save it bit by bit consciously. Although I had no idea when it would be of use, I always did it in earnest. Much know ledge about life acquired in childhood was passed on to us in this way.

As a child, I dried not only chenpi, but also chicken's gizzard – membrane which could cure dyspepsia. When I played with my friends who lived in the countryside, I could always find, laid out and dried in their courtyard were the flowers and plants picked from the farming land. They would tell me their names and what diseases they could cure respectively. What impressed me most was, one day I went to the home of a new friend, he took chance of the absence of the adults and showed me the poisonous scorpions kept in a big bamboo basket. All these medicines could be sold to help with the family budget. What's more, most of such labor was done by children. The playful things I did at the age of seven or eight, were unconsciously embedded in my memory of the traditional Chinese medicine.

In the 1970s, having gone through the socialist education and the movement of breaking the"four olds"(old ideas, old culture, old customs and old habits) , the majority of people who just became parents doubted that the folk prescription and empirical prescription could cure disease. Young parents who were thoroughly brainwashed would even take it as a shameful thing to believe traditional Chinese medicine was effective in treating illnesses. They dismissed TCM as something superstitious and unscientific. Living in such an urban environment, I failed to experience a more abundant traditional life style, which was a matter of regret for me. Just as all the treasure plants grow out from the earth, without the multi – layered and down – to – earth life experience, the human brain cannot foster wisdom in which school education plays only a limited part.

My friend brought genuine medicinal herbs

Several days ago, a friend of mine paid me a visit, bringing the treasures he sought out across the country which cost him half a year. He said these new treasures had brought him far more pleasure than the antiques, calligraphies and paintings he used to collect, so he decided to share them with me. It turned out that his new treasures were several common herbal plants which differed from others of the same kind only in quality, just like the striking difference between authentic West Lake Longjing Tea and the ordinary tea. Among the things he brought, there was Guangxi cassia twig(ramulus cinnamomi) which looked like the blood vessel. Its diameter, wall and the lumen all resemble human blood vessel and what's more, it has a strong unique smell. When smell it, Fengfu(an acupoint at the back side of the head) swells slightly and the blood seems to boil, one instinctively has an impulse to rise to his feet and stretch his arms. The shape and smell of Guangxi cassia twig are consistent with the medicinal effect of warming and clearing the blood vessel that cassia twig should have.

There is another herbal plant, the wild Chinese fevervine herb which takes the shape of the colon, whose cross section is exactly like the mucosal fold of the large intestine. The shapes of the mucous layer and muscle layer of the colon are vividly reflected in the cross section. Besides, its pipe diameter is similar to that of the colon, the smell of the herb marches into the lower abdomen, which stimulates the body to feel like defecating. The strong smell of the plant has such an impact on the qi and blood circulation of the human body that it suggests that the herb my friend sought out is genuine. The reason why my friend was so delighted is understandable. It is known that the amount of herbs needed and used is too large and that the yield of genuine herbs is limited in the geo – authentic producing areas, therefore the majority of herbs are not produced in the place of origin. Even if the herbs are grown in the place of origin, in order to improve production, farmers use a large amount of pesticides and fertilizers which make the quality of the

陈
皮
的
故
事

herbs declined. In addition, the harvesting time is not strictly controlled and there are some problems with the preservation, so the genuine herbs with high quality are practically rare, and the wild herbs are even rarer. If one is lucky to get some, no doubt he is wild with joy.

Why do genuine medicinal herbs have different curative effects? It's easy to understand, let's take grapes for example. Grapes grown in Turpan(Tulufan) , Xinjiang province are especially sweet while those of the same breed in other places are not. Present TCM doctors have one weak point, that is, their knowledge of the property of a medicine originates from books rather than practice. In most cases, they only know the names of medicinal herbs, but not their intrinsic properties of *Five Phases*, so they are very difficult to have a personal understanding of the roles of these herbs. This results in the fact that treating diseases and prescribing become a doctor's rearranging the descriptive words about the effects of the herbs instead of using the intrinsic properties of herbs to deploy a body – defending action. This kind of indirect intellectual experience is comparable to that a chef never knows what saltiness tastes but seasons food according to diners'tastes. Can you imagine that a chef who never tastes the flavors of seasonings is able to make delicious dishes under the guidance of the descriptive words? However, doctors currently trained by Chinese medical schools basically are like these chefs. I once advised my friend, one TCM lover, to have a personal experience of every medicinal herb and as a result, he gradually found that medicinal herbs which were available in hospitals or drugstores were too unreliable to achieve the desired effects recorded in ancient Chinese medical books. It is not that the descriptions on herbs in ancient books are wrong, but that the present medicinal herbs can' t guarantee their quality. So this conscientious friend began his journey looking for genuine herbs. The searching process brought him one surprise after another. The several bags of ordinary herbs must contain extraordinary stories and his happiness. He spent all afternoon to introduce his experience of looking for and how to distinguish genuine herbs and poor quality ones.

Xinhui Chenpi （tangerine peel）

My friend took out a bag of dried Xinhui chenpi of this year(tangerine peels produced in Xinhui city), whose color was like that of mandarin orange, green with yellow, just like the color of the peel after the flesh was just eaten by someone. The Chinese character"chen"means old. As the name suggests, the longer it is stored, the better curative effect it will have. Good chenpi has a deep color. And my friend's chenpi seems not to be that old, which doesn't have the dark look but looks more like the mandarin orange peel thrown away after the flesh being consumed. Though puzzled, I was all ears for my friend's account of the story. He said that this chenpi was purchased from a local medicinal herb grower. Originally he went to Xinhui, Guangzhou, with the intention to buy some best – quality chenpi. Impressed by his earnest attitude towards medicinal herbs, the grower told my friend the truth that chenpi available at the market which claimed to be stored for how many years is actually processed by technological means to look old. Having the appearance of the old tea, chenpi of this kind is actually not antique tangerine peel at all. As a matter of fact, it is very lucky to buy the genuinely local chenpi, because of the high demand and a limited yield of the local tangerine peels, the so – called local chenpi is mandarin orange peel shipped from other places and processed by dyeing. Later, the grower took my friend to his home, teaching him how to distinguish good chenpi. He told my friend if he really wanted old chenpi, he had to preserve the tangerine peel by himself because every year when the tangerine peel is in season, it is sold out immediately and there is no surplus of chenpi being kept in stock. What my friend told me enriched my knowledge of chenpi. The tangerine peel my friend brought is fresh, thus it has a color of yellowish green. Take a close look at chenpi, and one will find that its surface is covered with many small pores. Hold it up to the light and one can see there is a layer of oil droplets in the cortex and it's even more distinct where it's close to the pores, just as what human skin looks like under the magnifier. Put it close to the nostril and take a deep breath, one can feel the smell first sinks into the abdomen and shortly afterwards a fragrant smell emerges, soaring to the throat. The odor has rich layers and the prior smell and the latter fragrance are different, and also, which parts of the body they dwell in are varied. This rich odor conforms to the sinking and soaring characteristics of chenpi described in ancient Chinese medical books.

While chatting, I used half segment of one tangerine peel to make Kungfu Tea. It is said that if a prescription is tailored to the symptom, the medicine works as it passes down the throat. My consti-tution is characterized by phlegm dampness, therefore my voice is rather low and deep usually. After drinking two cups of tea, suddenly I felt my throat became dry. I knew the medicine worked. I cleared my throat and soon I real-

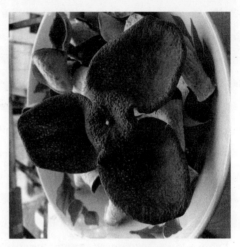

图 22 - 2 "新会陈皮"

ized that the same voice sounded brighter. And people around me perceived the change in my voice and we smiled at each other, overwhelmed with joy, for it proved that this chenpi was genuine medicinal herb.

My throat dried because the phlegm dampness accumulated there dispersed and cleared off. Accordingly, my voice naturally became clearer and brighter. This change is brought by the curative effect of chenpi, which is regulating qi, dissol-ving phlegm and clearing the throat. The fluid and humor of my body were driven to ascend by the hot tea of chenpi, so when I drank my fourth cup, the dryness in my throat turned into a soothing and refreshing feel and my body felt kind of brisk, too. This effect is given by the aftertast of Chenpi According to ancient Chinese, Chenpi has a heavy taste and light Qi , so the sinking and soaring prop-erties of chenpi have an attribute of yang within yin, and thus the fragrance odor can rise to the throat. If chenpi is baked in an oven, though nothing has changed in its appearance, the fragrant odor is destroyed by the drying function of the ov-en. As a result, its curative effect is weakened. Besides, the layer of oil is dried and dissipated. Without it, most medicinal properties of chenpi are lost accordingly. Though with the intact shape, the tangerine peel is absolutely not the medicinal herb called chenpi recorded in ancient medical books.

Everywhere on the earth, no matter whether it is human or a living being, without that qi, it is not the same being any more. Just as the saying goes, "man cannot do without his ambitions, a medicinal herb cannot work without its qi and an army cannot fight without the marshal." When it came to the way to acquire knowledge, ancient Chinese held that some people were born to know, they were superior; others learned to know, they were inferior. How did ancient Chinese know about the curative effect of chenpi? They had a wise learning technique called analogy and summary from nature.

The first distinctive feature of chenpi is that it is the peel of fruit, then it must have the general characteristic similar to the outer layers of all living things. The part of the body where chenpi works first has something to do with the outer layer. As for man, his skin that covers the body surface, the outer covering and the mucous membrane of his internal organs all fall into the category of outer layers. Take a close look at chenpi. Doesn't it particularly resemble human skin? It does not only have a surface of similar texture and evenly scattered pores, but also its outer layer is covered with a thin layer of oil. After aired and dried, if observed against the light, chenpi looks especially like animal leather and its structure is very similar to that of human skin under the magnifier. This is our impression of chenpi's outside surface.

It's more than that. Let's take a look at the internal surface of chenpi, which is nothing less than a perfect sample of human subcutaneous tissue: the white endothelium and the reticulate structure respectively correspond to the dermis and subcutaneous mucosa, in other words, interstices, or *couli* in terms of TCM. Chenpi is a entirety of epidermis and interstices. This gives us a big clue, that is, chenpi and human skin are similar at the information level, and thus, chenpi exerts some influence on the skin. But what on earth that influence can be like is determined by chenpi's characteristics of four qi and five "tastes". Therefore, the function acting on the skin is the pharmacological characteristic of chenpi. What's more, it is likely to be the fundamental function, the basis of all the other effects. Is that the case?

Tangerine pith

When eating a tangerine, one will find that there is a layer of tangling pith between the peel and the pulp. Like its peel, the tangerine pith is also a herbal medicine. The white pith spread over mainly between the segments and the peels, which is interconnected like a complex net. Its color and shape resemble the fascia that connects the internal organs and cavities of human body. This layer of fascia in the human body is called triple energizers fascia, the pathway of the original qi that travels across the five – zang viscera and six – fu bowels. Therefore, the dried tangerine pith acts on triple energizers fascia, while chenpi, the tangerine peel, tends to act on the epidermis. The two have similar medicinal properties but work on different parts of the body. Does this epidermis simply refer to the skin that covers the surface of the human body? Without doubt, it is more than that. The surfaces of all viscera and bowels are covered with a layer of epidermis called, in biological terms, serosa, which separates the organs from the surrounding areas of the cavities. Through this layer of epidermis, the five – zang viscera and six – fu bowels exchange energy and information with the surroundings. Chenpi can also work on the epidermis cells of these viscera and bowels. Besides the layer of serosa, the internal surfaces of such hollow organs as respiratory tract, gastrointestinal tract, even urinary bladder are covered with a monolayer of epidermis cells which are responsible for absorption and secretion, and also a gateway through which exchanges between the outside and inside of the organs can be done.

Life is based on exchange of substances between the internal and external environment, which is also the exchange of internal and external tissue cells. All the exchanges are achieved through the gateway of epidermis. Therefore, once there is an accumulation of the waste, the metabolism is affected. Where is this accumulation most likely to occur? There is no doubt that it occurs in the gateway where the exchanges are most frequently done.

The bitter taste, warm Qi and spicy smell of chenpi can clear and discharge the rubbish that adheres to the surface of the viscera and bowels, thus cleaning the pathway of substance and energy exchange between the inside and outside of the human body. This function of chenpi acting on the epidermis involves two kinds of cells, simple squamous epithelium and stratified squamous epithelium which cover all the viscera and bowels of the human body. Chenpi clears up the rubbish piling up at the gateway of all the organs. That's the exact reason why chenpi is used in TCM treatment of a wide range of diseases.

Ancient Chinese summarized the curative effects of chenpi, which include "regulating qi, dissolving phlegm, curing constipation and suppressing cough" when chenpi works on the epidermis of lungs and the large intestine, "stopping vomiting and uneasiness caused by empty stomach, regulating the spleen and the stomach, and stimulating the appetite"when it acts on epithelial cells of the gastrointestinal tract. As for another curative effect of chenpi, according to ancient Chinese, it is to"eliminate the residual heat and stagnant water from the urinary bladder". This effect is difficult to be understood by modern people. Let's make a careful analysis of it. The inside and outside layers of the urinary bladder are covered with mucous membrane and serosa if the gateways of these two layers are blocked up, then the exchange between the inside and outside of the urinary bladder is not smooth, which leads to the generation and build up of cold or heat that has the disfunction of the waterways. With the "analogy and summary from nature" method adopted by TCM, it's easily understood.

According to *Sheng Nong's Classic of Materia Medica*, the most authoritative canon of TCM, chenpi can benefit the absorption of water and food(the liquid nutrients) which are in essence the acquired qi that travels through the triple energizers fascia. Therefore, the benefit is actually to facilitate the flow of the triple energizers qi, and this coincides with the medicinal property of chenpi's inner surface together with the tangerine pith. If you cannot remember all of chenpi's curative effects, you just picture chenpi's playing the role of a servant who cleans the front gate of the high official's house with a broom in his hand. You will keep in mind all the curative effects of chenpi. In the Jin and Yuan Dynasty, a TCM doctor named Zhang Yuansu deemed that chenpi has the functions of"dumping, dispersing, harmonizing, warming, supplementing, dissolving phlegm and stopping cough, regulating the middle qi, strengthening the spleen and making the diaphragm agile, all these effects are superior to those of any other medicinal herbs".

Li Shizhen of Ming Dynasty made the comment, "chenpi can dump and dry due to its bitter taste, disperse with its pungent flavor, expert at treating all kinds of diseases."It's all due to the functions of chenpi of regulating qi and drying dampness. Therefore, chenpi cleans up the rubbish on one condition that there is a blockade at the gateway. If the gateway is unblocked, chenpi doesn't do any good, instead it consumes qi and blood.

Make good use of chenpi

In the QQ chat room of TCM lovers, there was such a thing happened. After learning about chenpi's medicinal properties, an enthusiastic mother immediately applied the knowledge into practice, making chenpi porridge for her child. Does this porridge really benefit the child? Don't forget that chenpi works only on the condition that there is an accumulation of rubbish within the body. Generally speaking, a child's body is not blocked up, and there is not so much fatty rubbish, so children usually reject the odor of chenpi. What is unacceptable to children includes not only chenpi, but also flavors of other foods many adults love, for instance, chili pepper, garlic, Chinese parsley, fennel, both white and black pepper etc. . The reason lies in the difference in constitutions. If a child likes a particular flavor, it suggests that there is some problem with the corresponding part of his or her body.

In food industry , the so – called qinghongsi, a special seasoning with a bright color and delicious flavor is made out of chenpi. The moon cake in my childhood had this seasoning. Why? Because the moon cake is rather oily, qinghongsi can clear up the gateway, keeping the exchanges smooth, and thus the epithelial tissues won't be stuck in the grease. Judging from the result, food with qinghongsi is easy to digest, and there will not be retention of food due to indigestion. Apart from the moon cake, when cooking food rich in fat and sugar, such as meat and the sweet rice with eight treasures, qinghongsi is used to promote absorption. If a person occasionally eats too much, he or she will suffer from abdominal distention and asthma. When this happens, drink some water boiled with chenpi to dissolve phlegm. And it will facilitate the circulation of qi and blood.

Do you know why fat people tend to die prematurely? It is because the rubbish within the body hinders the flow of the triple energizers'qi. Chenpi can clean up the rubbish and promote the flow of qi, in this perspective, so chenpi can help a person keep fit and live longer. Later doctors defined the medicinal properties of chenpi as"eliminating the stagnant qi", and if understanding it this way, we can't make full use of chenpi. Doctor Zhang Yuansu of the Song Dynasty interpreted the function of chenpi with"five abilities", that is, it can dump, disperse…and his interpretation of medicinal properties of chenpi is far more inclusive and better than that of many other doctors.

This respectable doctor, whoes another name is Zhang jiegu, is the founder of the theory of channel tropism of medicine herbs.

History of Xinhui chenpi

The famous Xinhui Chenpi is in fact not orange peel but tangerine peel. Xinhui Chenpi owed its popularity to a woman surnamed Mi from the Huang clan. 700 years ago during the reign of Emperor Lizong of the Song Dynasty, Queen mother Yang suffered from breast disease. Lady Mi, as an aristocratic lady, happened to attend the queen mother. She used the tangerine peel newly made in her home, located in Xinhui, to boil water for the queen mother to drink and it finally worked. After the queen mother recovered, Lady Mi was entitled"the First lady", the highest – ranking title for women at that time. After Lady Mi returned home when her service came to an end, she taught her clansmen to grow the tangerine trees and make the tangerine peel into the medicinal herb called chenpi. Since then, Xinhui Chenpi became world famous. And thus there was a new entry into the register of TCM recipes, called"Guang Chenpi"whose medicinal property was similar but stronger in curative effect, compared with the previous orange peel. Gradually, Guang Chenpi replaced the orange peel in TCM treatment. In the following centuries down to the Republic of China, the descendants of the Huang family unfailingly made and sold Guang Chenpi in Yinzhou Lake area and the lower reaches of Tanjiang River and Xijiang River. When at its peak, seven or eight out of ten households took up this business, creating a story of Guang Chenpi travelling around the world and taking the lead in the medicine market for 700 years.

陈
皮
的
故
事

(Second part)

The surface of chonpi is covered by a layer of on content, which the professionals think the more abundant, the quality of chenpi is better. Xinhui chenpi is well known for its oil content, which is higher than other production areas. Qi of water – food is the qi aequired after birth, which is integrated with qenuine qi and full of the body. If the qi of water – food is blaked by the airway, it may cause the swelling of phlegm – qi. Two conditions are required to eliminate the accumulated fat contents: one is to dissolve, the other is to push away. As we said in the previous chapter "Four Qi and five tastes", spicy causes dissipating heat and bitter causes dearing heat. The driving force of pushing comes from the spicy and bitter qi of chenpi, while the dissolution ability comes from the lil content which is contained by chenpi itself.

This is a little similar to what we have learned in the middle school chemistry – polar sdvent dissolves polar molecules, non – polar solvent dissolves mon – plar molecules. The chenpi with abundant oil content can dewmpose better the lily matters than attach on the epithelial layer, so it can eliminate the phlegm much better. Without that oil content, the spicy and bitter taste of becomes pure driving fore to operate qi, olny to disperse qi but not to eliminate the phlegm. It is just like the example that cleaning the oily bowl by water without dishwashiry detergent. Some people abvocate the use of Xinhui chempi water to prevent the pneumoconiosis caused by haze. The principle of eliminating the phlegm by chorpi is to clean up the garbage piled up in the portal through dissipation, purging and warming. The portal refers to the tissue epithe lium and cell membrane, and the waste eliminated ty chempi is from the accumulection qi of water – food, which is generated inside the body. Chenpi can cure vomiting and nausea caused ty the gastrointestinal waste, vomiting of water liquid, as well as spleen and lung phlegm – dampness clue to the deficienay of the spleen. This is the most appropriate way to use chenpi. However, dust particles in the hevze with in the scope of PM2. 5 is from the outside, this kind of particles accumulated in and between alveolus is not the qi of water – food, so drinking the chenpi water conld not dear up the clust partides sucked from the haze.

People may argue, for the same chenpi, why the longer, the expensive? what may change of chenpi's physical natures as time passing by? Yes, in different environment of space and time, the natures of any life change, but these changes are not obvious to the five senses. Fresh fruit just picked up from the tree tastes sour, and not delicious. Howerver, the taste chenges after keeping a period of time because the life of frait doesn't stop when it leaves the branch. In the storage phase. chenpi is still undergoing a chenge in a property. Any living creature is constantly exchanging information and energy with its surroundings. After the frost, the laste of persimmon becomes sweet, but after spring, it will not taste good any more, This is the offect caused by the change of the outside qifield on the persimmon. The taste of the pickle is better in the pickle jar half buried in the ground than that in the room of apartment, which is the effect of the earth qi on the pickle. The storge of chenpi is as same as the storage of tea, chenpi will continue to change in the following seasons affter the harvest. Accrading to the farmers who plant chenpi said, as winter in 2016 was not cold, the new chenpi this year was yellow – green, If the weather is very cold, the color of chenpi will become red, and the red chenpi tastes better.

The early taned chenpi has a wolrm characteristic and lacks mellow smell. After kept a long time, howerer, the taste will not be bitter and it smells mellow. As the thick smell and the oil content increase, the effect of elimiating phlegm, cleaning and warming properties are enhancing. Because the formen chenpi we have drunk described in the story part one has a short period of storage, we added some aeged ripe pu'er in it, hoping to achieve the effect of the old chenpi. Making tea of pu'er and chenpi together, actually contains the theory of water prcessing of chinese medicine. The ainghergsi (green red slice), which is made with orange peel, belongs to the proclssing category of traditional chinese medicine.

Similarly, after we drunk the chenpi tea that afternoon, a mother who lives in Jingzhou, Hubei province, sent a group of photos and text messages from QQ. Because her child ate a lot and caused excessive internal heet during the spring Festival, she let the child take thoree piecus of local smelly orange and the child recovered very soon. So she left me the message as follows:

陈
皮
的
故
事

1. All the local people says this kind of sour orange in Jingzhou as a good effect on eliminating the internal heat. Do you know this frant, Dr. zhang? It is better and sour.

2. Baidu says it is spicy, bitter and warm, and coneliminate the cold phlegm. But local people say it coneliminate the internal heat. If your lips are blistered or chapped, or your throat is uncomfortable, just eat three sour oranges. It is better than any other good medicines. This saying is different from Baidu. Is this kind of frait appropriate to both cold and hot symptoms?

3. People may have cold – heat complicated syndrome at the same time, but are there any double efficaey plants that can eliminate the cold and clear the heat?

4. Its academic name is found on Baidu. The smelly orange is a bit similar to pomelo. It is easy to distinguish between pemelos and smelly oranges. That is, the smelly oranges are smaller then the pomelos, and the epidermis of smelly oranges is a litte bit rougher thon the tangerine. The smelly oranges are bitter and sour, but the medical effect is quite good. Many people take them home, add honey to pickle and make the honey smelly oranges, which are very effective for the treatment of cough, phlegm and dredging. In Li Shizhen's lornpendium of Materia Medica of Ming dynasty, it recorded: "Good smelly orange is beneficial for qi circalation, reducing phlogm and curing cough. The effect is even better than the other medicines. The older the chenpi is, the better the treatment effect is." In Compendium of lompendium of Materia Medica of Qing Pynasty, it recorded, "The smelly orange can cure phlegm disease, eliminate the fat, improve digestion, help to sober up and regalate qi and detoxicate crab poison."

This mother is also on amateur of traditional chinese medicine. After eating three smelly oranges, her child was recoverd from saffering overfeeding and excessive internal heet. She was so happy and surprised that she would like to communicate with me as showed above. I told her that she got to know a good herb when she returned home this time. The smelly orange should be a kind of medicinal materid, just as Xinhui chenpi. Therefore, I suggest her collect some smelly oranges and take back to shenzhen, preferably pickled with honey. The smelly orange can help the digestion and eliminate the phlegm. It is beneficial for those children who are prone to overfeeding, and also for those adults with heavy phlegm to cleam up the phlegm and indigestion.

The smelly orange is to clear up excessive fire in gastrointestinal tract ceeused by eating too much meat. Because of its spiciness and bitterness, it can help eliminate the blocks in intestines. As the excessive fire of the gastrointestinal tract goes down, the child's symptoms of exassive internal heat are gone away. It is not tree that the smelly orange cannot eliminate the internal heat because of its warm nature. Here are the treatment method we use is not to cure the heat by the cold, but to eliminate garbage in order to make the stomach and intestines harmonious and comfortable. If there is no garbage in the stomach and intestines, eating smelly orange will arouse internal heat, because the worm nature of smell orange may make more normal body fluid and humor out of the body, especially for these children of deficient body fluid and hamor. Therefore, TCM cloctors stress providing the correct herbs ofter the proper diagnosis, and stopping the medicine as the disease is cured.

The medical problems that this mother encountered show that there is no absolute good or bad herb in the world. It is beneficial if we use wisely, and harmful if we use wrongly.

The use of tangerine peel

There is another famous tangerine peel produced in HuaZhou city, Guangdong Province, known as "Huazhou red tangerine peel", and the characteristic of best chenpi are big and thin peel, orange red, oily matter and many white tangerine piths. Why is that?

The principle is the same as Xinhui chenpi, but Huazhou red tangerine peel has more pubescence, so its shape looks more closer to the skin of human. Lung governs skin, so Huazhou red tangerine peel has a better curative effect to lung phlegm than other kinds of chenpi.

Why is the highest grade chenpi considered with lots of oily matter? Because the damp phlegm of human body always includes oil. The oil on chenpi can guide it's clean – up function.

The striking effect of chenpi is to regulate the flow of Qi and eliminate the phlegm. There is a famous prescription that can eliminate the phlegm, called *Two - chen decoction*. It is very suitable for morden pepole who have phlegm - dampness constitution but with less physical excises. It also can cure modern diseases what caused by phlegm - dampness constitution, such as hyperlipidemia, hyperglycemia and arthropathy.

This prescription is made of pinellia ternata, tangerine peel, poria cocos and radix liquiritiae. It can eliminate dampness and reduce phlegm and keep the qi circulating in the body and alleviate disease. It is the basic prescription of treating cold - dampness and reducing phlegm. Grind fourherbs into powder. Every time take ten gram power and add multiple pieces of fresh ginger and a dark plum. Water decoction of these herbs are decocted by water and one patient has warm - taken without eating drug residues.

If the damp phlegm is accumulated in stomach and intestines, then the stomach qi rises with nausea and vomiting. If the damp phlegm is accumulated in chest and diaphragm, then qi is obstructed with chest and the stomach is discomforted. If the damp phlegm is accumulated in lung, then appears phlegmy throat and cough, together with the bowel movement impeded. If the damp phlegm impedes qi running in the triple energizer meridians, then appears the phlegmatic hygrosis and the dizziness. If the phlegm blocks heart, then there appears the palpitation, pale face, heart deficiency and suspicion. This is because face can tell us whether or not the heart is well. If the phlegm blocks the muscles of spleen, then heavy limbs appears.

Tangerine peel is bitter and pungent so it can excrete phlegm - dampness outside the body. Poria cocos can dispel water - dampness. This prescription works through eliminating the phlegm, retaining fluid and water - damp pathological matters. Pinellia ternata is dry so it can eliminate dampness and phlegm. Tangerine peel is bitter and pungent so it can reduce phlegm. It is required that the pinellia ternata and dried tangerine peel should be stored for a long time. Therefore this prescription is also called"*Two Chen Soup*". The combination of pinellia ternata and tangerine peel is common in the phlegm - expelling formula to regulate qi and reduce the phlegm.

In the *Two Chen decoction*, the yellow, thick and pungent fresh ginger can help pinellia ternata and dried tangerine peel to reduce phlegm, because the essence of fresh ginger can be absorbed by stomach and lung, which promotes the Qi movement of lung and stomach and further promotes the Qi operation of water – food essence. If the damp phlegm is accumulated in stomach, fresh ginger is necessary. *JinKuiYaolue(Synopsis of Prescriptions of the Golden Chamber, authored by Doctor Zhongjing Zhang, 3C CHN)* wrote a classic prescription which used the combination of dried tangerine peel and fresh ginger to treat abnormal flow of stomach qi, through dispelling exopathogens with pungent and promoting the circulation of qi. When the prescription of ginger – pinellia ternata decoction, added with ginger juice, is used, the pungent – dispersing quality of fresh ginger is greatly enhanced. When added with several dark plums, the prescription can prevent impairment of body fluid which results in excessive internal heat.

Other uses of the *Two Chen Decoction*:

It can be used to treat the damp phlegm by adding rhizoma atractylodis and Mangnolia officinalis to increase the ability to dry the dampness and reduce the phlegm.

It can be used to treat the heat phlegm by adding rhizoma arisaematis (cum bile) and Gualou to clear the heat and eliminate the phlegm.

It can be used to treat the cold phlegm by adding dry ginger and asarum to warm the cold phlegm.

It can be used to treat wind – phlegm dizziness by adding gastrodia tue and stiff silkworm to eliminate the phlegm and calm the wind.

It can be used to treat the food phlegm by adding radish seed and malt to promote digestion and eliminate the phlegm.

It can be used to treat the stagnated phlegm by adding rhizoma cyperi, pericarpium citri reticulatae viride and curcuma to lift the depression and resolve the phlegm.

It can be used to treat the crewels and phlegm nodes when the phlegm blocks the Qi channels, by adding seaweed, kelp and oyster to soften the hardness and eliminate the phlegm.

End story of tangerine peel.

论咸味

On salty taste

中国有句古话叫做"好厨子一把盐"，意思是盐使用得恰到好处，饭菜可以变得更加可口。但是这个观点现在受到了另一种流行健康观念的挑战，就是清淡饮食可以保健康，这种观念认为吃过多的盐可以引起包括高血压在内的多种慢性疾病。这种说法如果成立，咸味就可能成了一种致病因素，与我们所说的五味营养观相矛盾。那么咸味对人体健康到底有没有危害呢？让我们从头细说。

人为什么离不开盐？

在中医营养观里我们已经知道，五味对应人体五行五藏，所以口味的选择，来自于人身体天然调节机制。咸味是五味之一，对咸味的需求，也是由人体五藏功能的决定。盐不仅是厨房里最重要的调味品，而且是维持健康不可缺少的食材。

盐曾经是人类社会最重要的自然资源，这个资源对人类社会的影响超过了其他任何天然的资源。直到今天，盐的生产销售仍然是被控制的。中国上古历史上有一场对中华民族影响最大的战争，黄帝蚩尤之战，就与争夺对盐资源的控制有关。

有人认为动物可以不额外吃盐而存活，所以人也可以离开食盐而生存。这源于不了解人与动物的身体差异。人和动物最大的区别是：人的肉体羸弱而大脑强大，动物有强悍的肉身却不擅思考。所以在人看来，动物的生命力特别顽强。俗话说"猫有九条命"就是这个意思。

人自称为万物之灵，原因在于人的脑力发达、善于思考，所以成为了现阶段地球的主宰者。肾主骨生髓，脑为髓海，大脑的思维活动，来自于肾精和肾气。人的思维活动越旺盛，越消耗肾精肾气。肾精是人的先天之本，肾气是人体生命的原动力，肾"精"是人体先天之本，主宰寿命。肾气和肾精的大量消耗，导致人类大脑发达而肾气弱。肾气弱则肉体相对于动物就显得羸弱，动物没有强大的思考能力但是肾气足肉身强大。我们会发现动物运动时多是或跑或跳，非常轻健敏捷，而人则相对迟慢。与动物相比，人的身体更容易生病而且很难活到正常的寿命，直接原因与大脑对肾精和肾气的消耗有关。尤其是无序散乱的思维活动最耗费人的肾精和肾气。生活经验告诉我们，越是容易胡思乱想的人，肾气越弱，身体也就越差，思虑过重甚至会导致夭折。

那么人是不是要拒绝思考呢？当然不是，因为造物主对人的最初设计即不同于动物，所以停止思考是不可能的。即便是一个狼孩，只要有外因的触动，他仍然会使用大脑，这是基因决定的。既然人不可能避免思考，那么就看怎样思考了。东方上古圣人发现人的思考只要专注和符合逻辑，对肾气的损耗可以降到最小。所以中国古代的养生家主张起居、饮食、劳作合于道，思想行为越合乎逻辑越能保持健康。如果配合以动作和呼吸，甚至可以反过来培植肾精肾气，令其更充盈。所以他们创造了围绕"气"的身心修炼方法，不但强身健体，甚至可以弥补先天不足，这就是东方养生学。

肾、肝、脑与体能、动作和思想的关系

肾藏精主骨生髓，髓生肝，肝主人体之筋膜，筋膜为元气之通道，又主关节强弱灵活及承受力。所以肾气充沛，髓海丰盈则筋膜强健，故肉身强大。脑为髓之海，髓海有余，则轻劲多力，髓海不足则双目无神，懈怠安卧。和动物行动比较会发现"懈怠安卧"是指■人日常状态最传神的一个词语。

五藏六腑之精气，皆上于目而为睛，骨之精为瞳子，筋之精为黑眼，血之精为络。故从人的眼神可以观察到他的健康状态。倘若思虑杂乱，相当于髓海里出现了一个地沟，肾气都沿着地沟漏掉啦，那么眼神就是涣散无力的。伍子胥过韶关一夜白头的故事，就是思虑过重肾气一夜之间耗散所致。常常见有的人因为巨大的精神压力消耗肾精肾气，一夜之间老了很多岁，体现了忧思忧虑对身体的影响。

因为大脑发达，消耗大量肾精肾气身体的肾精肾气相对与动物就会显得不足，肉身虚弱就容易生病。为了弥补这个缺陷，人创造了御寒方法和一日两餐的生活习惯，从此有了对衣服和住宅的需求。

因为人类的肾气相对弱，为了维持正常活动，就需要盐来提升肾气就好像炉膛的火力不足，需要用扇子扇火一样。而动物不因脑力消耗大量肾精肾气，一般食物已足以维持生命活动所需，通常不需额外摄入盐分。所以民间有"一咸三分味"的说法。

不仅如此，因为人的肉体虚弱，对食物的消化吸收能力也减弱，动物可以直接取用草木果实血肉，而人需要吃熟食来弥补机能的缺陷。所有食物当中，谷物气味最平和，所以选择了五谷作为主食。为了濡养相对羸弱的身体，还需要配合以五菜、五果和五畜，以火烹饪，佐以调料来滋养人体的五藏系统，令其维持平衡。所以，《内经》中说人的饮食必须："五谷为养，五果为助，五畜为益，五菜为充，气味合而服之，以补精益气"。

其次人类还需要食盐和各种调味品来调节五藏之气的平衡，是为"五味调和"。所以就有了酸甜苦辣咸各种调味品的使用，由此形成了人类特有的饮食文化。同样重量的食物中，肉类所含的能量高于谷物，谷物又高于大多数水果，食物的能量越密集，消化所需要消耗的元气越多，所以做肉食通常要放更多的盐，而水果可以直接生吃。谷物介于二者之间。

说咸味

五味之中的咸味可以入肾以激发肾中元气升腾，肾中元阳相当于煮饭时锅底的火，没有这把火，中焦的水谷就不能腐熟，将水谷精华上腾于上焦心肺。所以人类需要盐来维持肾气的升腾。

生活中我们会发现一个规律，就是年龄越小，对咸味的需求越低，年龄越大口味越重。肾气越弱越嗜盐，身体越通畅，对盐的需求量越少。老年人肾精肾气下降，为了维持五藏正常功能，作为身体本能反应，需要通过摄入更多的咸味以增加肾气，来维持生命机能。所以老年人嗜盐，是肾气不足导致的生理反应，为身体纠偏之举。

中医认为肾气是一身元气之本。肾气不足，轻一点的表现为体力和精力下降，记忆力衰退，包括免疫力和修复力的降低。重一点的则表现为有形疾病，比如高血压、心脏病。大多数的老年病都与肾气衰退有关，所以解决问题的关键是如何保存和恢复肾气。而且对肾气的保护是从未病阶段就开始的，而不是等到了发病阶段才控制盐的摄入量，防患未然，这就是中医特有的养生之法。

在中医里，老年病是指由于肾气衰退导致的机能下降和由此产生的生理变化。但现状是，很多不属于老年性疾病的患者也嗜好咸味，这是因为生活方式不节导致的阴阳失衡、痰饮水湿堆积和气血瘀滞。当身体内痰饮水湿堵塞了经脉，那么元气运行就需要更大的动力方能冲破阻碍来完成向全身供给能量的任务，这个动力从哪里来？还是自肾中而来，就好像锅炉管道阻塞就要消耗更多的燃料才能完成蒸汽供给一样。所以有此类疾病的人亦偏向于嗜好咸味，来激发肾气。由此可见不论是年龄导致的肾精不足还是病理产物堆积造成的经脉不通，都会出现嗜好咸味的症状，对于此类病人一味地控制食盐量，会阻碍身体自主恢复机制。部分老年人的精力不济和血压增高是肾气不足直接或间接导致的结果，所以他们会出现嗜咸的表现。非食盐导致了高血压，而是因为肾精不足肾气减弱，同时导致了嗜盐和高血压。

除咸味之外，辛味是排位第二的调味品，辣椒、胡椒、花椒、八角、大料、芥末和葱姜蒜都属于辛味。细胞所需要的营养是水谷精微和肺气化合而成的，肺最容易被寒邪封闭造成肺活量下降，辛味可以驱寒开表，增加肺气的力量。所以常食辛味可以增加肺气，进而起到养生保健作用。

民以食为天，饮食文化是人类文化集大成者，好中医如果升级一下，就是好厨子。好厨子再懂了山医命卜相的学问，就是养生家了。

味觉识健康

心主神明，为君主之官。自主选择口味，本身就是身体自我调整的一种本能。如果违背"心"意勉强坚持清淡饮食或者忌口，其实就是阻止了身体的自我调整。所以违背心意坚持忌口的人，其实并不会因此单一原因而改善健康，那么是不是应该喜好什么就吃什么呢？答案并不绝对，口味的嗜好，是人体发出的一个信号。在从食物到化生营卫气血再到细胞的利用这个过程中任何生理功能的异常，都会导致口味甚至食量的改变。所以口味嗜好是身体表现出来的需求，这个需求既有可能是真正的缺少，也可能是消化吸收以及运输环节上的异常，所以需要对口味嗜好做更细致的分析。

不是因为口味改变引发了疾病，而是五藏不调导致了口味嗜好的变化。所有疾病在早期是隐藏不显的，但口味的变化最容易被发现。所以从一个人口味的偏好，可以推断五脏虚实而给予对症治疗，中医的诊断和治疗是统一在五行能量层面的。

There is an old Chinese saying to describe the importance of salt control for a cook, "The proper salt makes an excellent cook". This means that proper addition of salt can make the dishes more delicious. But today this view of salt is facing the challenge of another popular health concept which advocates that light diet can keep people healthy. They regard that eating much salt will cause many chronic diseases including hypertension. If that's the case, salty taste may be a pathogenesis of diseases. This conflicts with the nutriology view of five tastes. Is the salty taste really harmful to human health? Let's talk about it from the very beginning.

Why people cannot live without salt?

We've got some knowledge from Chinese traditional medicine that the *five tastes* are corresponding to the *five phases* and to the *five – zang temples*. Which taste to choose depends on the body natural regulation mechanisms. Salty taste is one of the *five tastes*. The demand of salt also depends on the functions of the five – zang temples. Salt is not only the most important condiment in kitchen but also the indispensability food stuff to keep people in health.

Salt used to be the most important natural resource in human society. The influence of salt is much more than any other natural resources. Until today, the manufacturing and selling of salt are still under control. In the ancient times in China, there was a battle which had a huge impact on the Chinese nation and happened between the Yellow Emperor and Chiyou for the control on salt resources.

Some people regard that animals can live without salt, so does the mankind. They do not know the body differences between human beings and animals. The biggest difference is that human beings have weak physical bodies with developed brains, while animals have strong bodies but with less thoughts. So mankind regards that animals are of great vitality, just as the Chinese saying goes that a cat has nine lives.

Human beings consider themselves as the wisest creatures, because they have developed brains which are good at thinking and can make them to be the current masters on the earth. The kidney dominates the bone and marrow, and the brain is the sea of marrow. All the brain activities energy is from the kidney essence and qi. The deeper one falls in overthinking, the more kidney essence and qi will be consumed. Kidney essence is the root of life, and kidney qi is the driving force of life and they are in charge of longevity. Over – consumption of kidney essence and qi will make the brain stronger but make qi insufficient. Compared with animals, human body is weaker. On the contrary, animals cannot think precisely but they have strong physical bodies under the support of full kidney qi. We find that animals always run fast or jump quickly and lightly, but people are reatively slow. Mankind is easier to be attacked by diseases. Therefore, it is difficult for mankind to live to a maturated age. The direct reason of early death is that the exhaustion of kidney essence and qi consumed by brain activities, especially by disordered thoughts. Based on the experience in daily life, one's kidney qi will be weaker if he always takes himself into disordered thoughts. His body will be worse, too. Overthinking can lead one to pre – maturated death.

Shall people stop thinking to reserve their kidney essence and qi? Of course not. It is impossible for mankind to stop thinking because mankind becomes different from animals in the evolution process. Even a wolf – child can use his brain to think when an external accident occurs to him. Man's thinking ability is decided by genes. This design requests mankind to use brain to think. It is impossible to avoid thinking, and the next question for people is how to think. The ancient Chinese sages had found that one could minimize the consumption of kidney qi if he concentrated his attention and put his thoughts in logic. The ancient sages who focused on health prevention also advocated that all mankind's activities in daily life should follow the *Tao*, rising and resting, drinking and eating regularly. The more logical one's thinking and doing are, the heathier his body is. Proper exercises and breath practice can supplement one's kidney essence and qi to make them more abundant. Based on the extensive research, ancient sages invented a practice method of qi. This practice method can not only keep physical body in health, but also make up for congental deficienly. This is the oriental classic philosophy of health preservation.

Relationships between kidney, liver and brain, and physical energy, behavior and thoughts

The kidney reserves the essence, dominates the bone, and engenders the marrow. Then the marrow engenders the liver, the liver nourishes the tendons and fascia. The tendons and fascia are the channels of source qi in a body. They are related to the flexibility and capability of joints. So both the tendons and physical body will be stronger if the kidney qi is sufficient. If the kidney qi is abundant, and the marrow sea is full, then the tendons and fascia are strong, and the physical body is powerful. This is good chain actions for body. The brain is the sea of marrow. One will be active and powerful if the marrow is full. On the contrary, if the marrow is insufficient, one will become lazy to lie with soulless eyes. Lying Lazily is the most appropriate word to describe mankind in present daily life.

The essence of both five – zang temples and six – fu bowels concentrates upward to the eyes. The bone essence is embodied in pupil, and the tendons essence is embodied in black eye, and the blood essence is embodied in collaterals. Therefore, we can judge whether one is healthy by observing his eyes. If one's thoughts are in disorder, as like a trench occurs in his marrow sea. The kidney qi will be leak away through the trench. Then the look in his eyes will scatter due to the leakage of kidney qi. There is a historical story about the overthinking influence on the kidney qi. Zixu Wu's hair turned white in one night before he broke through the barriers in Shaoguan. There are also many other people who become older in one night because of big pressure. These stories indicate that overthinking and worrying really can damage the kidney qi and finally damage the physical body.

Human beings have developed brains, which consume lots of kidney essence and qi, thus their kidney essence and qi of body are less abundant than animals. Their bodies are not as stronger as animals. Diseases can invade human bodies easily. To make up for this defect of weak body, pople had to create some methods and form a diet habit with two – meal one day. Hereafter people have the demand for doths and houses.

In order to keep all activities normally, people must eat salt to fortify their kidney qi, just like the small fire in hearth meeds to be fanned. But the animals can live well without thinking too much. So normal food without extra salt can make ends meet. Salt is the necessary food stuff for mankind, as the saying goes that "Salty is the basic one among all the five tastes. "

Meanwhile, mankind's digestion and absorption ability are weaker due to the intrinsically weak bodies. The animals can eat food directly, such as grass, trees, fruits, blood, meat. But human beings always need to eat the cooked food to make up their functional defect on digestion and absorption. Among all food, the grain is the mildest and softest food. People finally choose the five grains as their main food. They need to cook food with fire, adding condiments. The cooked foods of five vegetables, five fruits and five animals can nourish the five – zang temples, and keep them in balance. Therefore, a suitable diet structure is mentioned in the *Yellow Emperor's Classic of Medicine*. The five grains are used to nourish, the five fruits to assist, the five animals to fortify, the five vegetables to fulfill. Combining the energetic properties of these in one's diet can reinforce the essence and qi. People also need salt and kinds of condiments to balance the qi in the five – zang temples. It is the harmony among five tastes. Later, all kinds of condiments, such as sour, sweet, bitter, hot and salty, are used in the meals, And thus the unique diet culture came into true. Among the same weight of foods, the energy in meat is more than grain, energy in grain is more than that in fruits. The more energy a food stuff has, the more source qi will be consumed for digestion. So the demand of salt is different for different foods. It depends on the energy in food. More salt is needed for meat, less for grains. The fruits can be eaten without salt, without cooking.

论
咸
味

The Salty Taste

The Salty taste pours into the kidney, stimulating the source qi to ascend. The yuan yang(innate Yang) in kidney is like the fire under the cooking pot. The water and food in pot cannot be boiled if the fire is small. Similarly, the water and the grains in middle energizer cannot be digested timely without yuan yang in kidney and, the essence of food cannot be transported upward to the heart and lung in the upper energizer.

We've found a rule that the younger like light taste diet, the older like heavy taste food. If one's kidney qi is deficient, he prefers to heavy salty taste. On the contrary, one needs less salt if he has a strong body. The older needs more salt to reinforce the kidney qi to maintain the functions of the five – zang temples when the kidney essence and qi decline. It is the natural response of life. Heavy salty taste is the auto – corrective actions of body itself when the kidney qi is deficient.

It is considered that the kidney qi is the root of source qi in traditional Chinese medicine. When one's kidney qi is deficient slightly, both his physical and metal energy will descend, his memory will deteriorate gradually, his immunity and recovery ability will decline accordingly. When one's kidney qi is deficient seriously, the diseases will occur, such as hypertension and heart disease. Most of the aged diseases are connected to the decline of kidney qi. The key point to avoid disease is to keep and recover the kidney qi. People should protect the kidney qi well before diseases invade body instead of control the salt until he is ill. This is the particular way of Chinese classic health preservation.

In traditional Chinese medicine the aged diseases are the physiological change caused by kidney qi declination and its weakened functions. In fact, many patients who do not have the aged illness also like heavy salty taste. Their irregular life styles result in the imbalance of *ying* and *yang*, retention of water, dampness, phlegm, stagnation of qi and blood. When the channels and collaterals are blocked by water, phlegm and dampness inside, The source qi needs more power to break through the blockages, then to provide energy to the whole body. Where does the power derive from? It is from the kidney. It is like the boiler needs more fuel beneath to produce enough steam to break through when the boiler pipe is blocked. Such patients also like heavy salty taste to stimulate their kidney qi.

These patients prefer to heavy salty taste whatever their kidney qi is insufficient coming with age, or their channels are blocked due to stagnation of pathological things. Salt – restricted diet on such patients will prevent their bodies from self – recovery mechanism running. Some elderly people often feel less energetic and have hypertension. This is directly or indirectly caused by the insufficiency of his kidney qi. After they have this feeling, the elderly start to prefer to heavy salty diet. It doesn't the salt lead to the blood pressure high but the insufficiency of kidney essence and qi does, and which changes the taste into salty preference, at the same time.

Besides salt, pungent is the second flavor in daily popular condiments. All kinds of pepper belong to pungent condiments, such as hot peppers, white/black peppers, Sichuan peppers, star anise, aniseeds, and mustard. Onions, gingers and garlics are all pungent condiments, too. The nutrition of cells is the combination of water – food essence with the lung qi. The capacity of lung will become smaller when the cold – evil invades the lung. At this moment, pungent can be used to open the pores in skin and expel the cold – evil. Pungent taste can promote the power of lung qi. It can be used as a method of health preservation and care.

Food is the first necessity of mankind. Diet culture epitomizes the human culture. A professional doctor of traditional Chinese medicine can turn to be a good cook, then grow up to be an expert on health preservation if he has some knowledge of divination.

To predict one's health from his favorite taste.

The heart temple is the monarch of all the five ones, which is in charge of one's consciousness. Which taste to choose is the instinctive function of body. It is decided by the heart according to the body's actual demand. Disobeying the heart to insist the light diet or refuse the certain food is actually prevent the body from adjusting itself. One will fail to improve his health only by refusing the certain food. Another question comes. Should one eat whatever he likes? No, it is not absolutely. The choice of taste is a signal of body. It is a complete process that the food is digested to produce nutritive qi and defensive qi, then to be used by cells. During this process, every abnormal functions will change the taste, or even change the appetite. Which taste to choose is the actual demand manifested by body. It may be the real shortage of body, or may be the abnormal manifestation in the digestion and transition process. We need to analyze the root cause in more details.

It is not taste change but the inharmony of five – zang temples to cause diseases. The diseases hide inside at the beginning. It is difficult to be felt at this time. But the patient's taste change can be easily found. A doctor of traditional Chinese medicine can predict the deficiency and excess of five – zang temples according to patient's taste change. In traditional Chinese medicine, the diagnosing and treating diseases are analyzed on the same energy level of the five phases.

营气与卫气

Nutrient Qi and Defensive Qi

摄入食物并把食物中的能量还原出来，是人体从外界获取能量的一个主要渠道。固态食物进入消化道，逐步消化分解为可以穿透肠黏膜的微粒，这个过程是由人体的消化和吸收系统来完成的。从口腔、胃到大小肠通过消化道黏膜壁吸收人体内的微粒，称之为水谷精微。水谷精微可理解为是变得细小的食物微粒，它要被全身的组织细胞使用，还需要一个变化和运输的过程，这个过程需要肺的呼吸和血脉的参与。所以人体有效能量的灌注，不仅仅是食物的消化吸收，还与呼吸和血运有关。

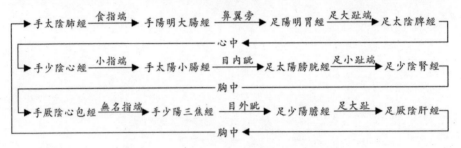

图25-1 营气循行手足阴阳十二经详图

现代生理学研究显示，人体胃对食物的排空时间是4-6小时，就是说食物进入胃之后，通过胃的消化变为食糜，然后送入小肠继续消化吸收，这个过程需要四个小时。这就意味着一个饥饿的人现在开始吃饭，四小时以后他身体才能补充到能量而恢复体力。但实际情况不是这样的。饥肠辘辘的人，只要给他一碗饭，饭一下肚立刻能感受到体力的恢复，而实际上此刻他的肚子还并没有吃饱。

一个人运动大汗之后口渴难耐，这时候需要喝水来补充水分。如果一大杯凉水喝下去，会觉得非常爽快。但是问题来了，过了不久继续感觉口渴，所以需要不断地喝水。喝凉水解渴，会喝下去很多水；另外一种情况就是喝少量的热水，大家会有这种体会，喝热水只需要很少量，不但解渴而且解乏，这是为什么呢？原来人体对能量的需求，即有物质的一面又有动力的一面。这两方面共同为生理活动提供支持，这就是中医里水谷如何转化为营气和卫气的理论。

五藏六腑系统

前几章的论述，我们已经知道"五藏"是一个来源于能量模型系统的虚拟概念。但人又是一个物质体，所以必须有相应的实体来完成物质代谢功能。完成食物消化吸收转运功能的是人体的六腑系统，完成五藏调解功能的是实体的心肝脾肺肾五脏系统，它们共同构成人体五藏六腑系统，以经脉连接起来。五藏系统与实体解剖的心肺肝脾肾，六腑系统与实体解剖的小肠、大肠、三焦筋膜、胆、胃、膀胱有对应吻合之处。

营气的生成

食物被消化分解为水谷精微，通过胃肠道的黏膜上皮进入到小肠壁内血管和淋巴管之中，层层汇聚，最后通过腔静脉和胸导管汇集进入心脏再上输于肺。由此看出，全身的组织细胞并没有直接使用从肠道而来的水谷精微，而是先输入了心脏，再由心脏至肺，与肺中的空气化合。这个由食物到水谷精微的过程，由胃、小肠、大肠、三焦、膀胱共同参与完成。胃主腐熟受纳，小肠主受盛，大肠管传导，胆主调节，膀胱气化水液、三焦通调水道。六腑的协同作用将水谷精微上输与肺，水谷精微与肺中的空气化合而生成营气，通过血液循环灌注全身，被组织细胞利用。由此可见，人体营气的质量，不但与摄入的食物有关，还与肺内空气的质量以及充足度相关。

营卫辨析

食物进入胃中，其所带的能量最终分为两部分，化为营气的清气部分和化为卫气的浊气部分。浊者其性慓疾滑利，可以迅速散入人体，行于脉外，称为卫气，所以卫气能快速充溢于人体。热水和凉水的区别是较高的温度增加了水饮中的滑利彪悍之气，可以迅速扩散，所以解渴的效果更好。饮食中的浊气成分也可以入胃即扩散于体内，故热食和烹制的辛散鲜香的食物，对人体更有利。卫气特点是加强组织细胞自身的功能，能温养一身脏腑，滋养腠理，护卫肌表，开阖汗孔，防御外邪。营气是物质性营养成分。打一个比方，如果要新建一座城市，既需要工匠又需要建筑材料，那么卫气就相当于工匠，营气就相当于通过铁路运送的建筑材料。营气回流入血脉之中，通过血管运输到五脏六腑，以荣四末，故营气运行于脉中，卫气运行于脉外，这是水谷化为人体营卫之气，为全身细胞提供能量的过程。倘若营卫之气不足，那么五脏机能、抵抗力、精神意志都会比较偏低。这就是营卫与人体生命的关系。

既然剽悍滑利之气是卫气的来源，那么气味浓烈带有刺激性气味的食材就可以生成更多的卫气，黏腻厚重的食材可以产生更多的营气，大枣和生姜可以看做生成营卫之气的两个代表物，不仅如此，一切具有浓烈气味的调味品都可以看做是增加卫气的食料。营气和卫气是一对阴阳关系，他们之间需保持平衡关系才能保证健康。营气虚卫气盛，或卫气虚营气盛都会造成疾病。这提示我们不论饮食营养还是药物配比，都要注意营卫之气的协调，卫气偏盛则耗气，营气偏盛则粘滞。故内经说"五脏坚固，血脉和调，肌肉解利，皮肤致密，营卫之行，不失其常，呼吸微徐，气以度行，六腑化谷，津液布扬，各如其常，故能长久"。

营卫之气的运行规律

卫气的基本循环规律是白昼清醒时行于阳，黑夜入眠行于阴。可以理解为眼睛一睁卫气就外出，然后人开始了各种工作，眼睛一闭卫气就入内，卫气行于阴，是从足少阴经注于肾，而后至心、肺、肝、脾，复还于肾。从这个特征可见，卫气对内脏的濡养修复是在睡眠中进行的，睡眠的重要性就在于此，人在睡眠当中五藏系统得到卫气的濡养和调整，这就是长期睡眠不足会导致生病的原因。

体表皮肤是人体的防御前线．睡眠中卫气入里，假如一个人睡着后没有盖被子，皮肤表层卫气不足，风寒就容易乘虚而入导致感冒。

营气的运行空间和时间规律是这样的，平旦寅时，从手太阴之寸口始，自手太阴注手阳明，足阳明注足太阴，手少阴注手太阳，足太阳注足少阴，手厥阴注手少阳，足少阳注足厥阴，足厥阴注手太阴，周而复始。

六腑运化食物而成水谷精微，水谷和肺之清气而生成人身之营气，营气运行于脉管之内，脉管中的血液，充当了营气的载体，营养五脏六腑，四肢末节，属于人体物质营养的循环通道。营气要被组织细胞所用，必须先透脉管壁，渗入到组织间隙，再通过细胞膜进入细胞内部才能发挥滋养作用。这个过程叫做人体的微循环。

营气的时间性运行规律提示我们，微循环的开放与时间相关。微循环的强弱与组织的生理功能以及防御修复相关。比如辰时营气过胃经，那么意味着此时胃经系统所属的组织器官处于微循环开放活跃阶段，是一天当中消化吸收能力最强的时候，就好像太阳上午照东窗，下午照西窗，时间不同，所受阳光会有差异。营气的时间运行特征在养生保健上令我们脑洞大开，由此产生了中医里与时间有关的健身和治病方法。比如营气运行旺于肝经时，肝经所调控的微循环开放，肝经所属的解毒藏血功能最强。

中医生命结构观

人体六腑的作用是将食物分解转化为水谷精微，并转运水谷精微、同时将食物中的代谢废物排出体外，六腑运输的水谷精微在心肺两脏化生为营气和卫气，营卫之气的运行道路为人体经脉，那么五藏的作用是什么呢？中医认为人的生命层次有物质层面和更高级的非物质层面，五藏主管人的精神和意识活动。

《黄帝内经》言："人之血气精神者，所以奉生而周于性命。

经脉者，所以行血气而荣阴阳，濡筋骨，利关节者也。

卫气者，所以温分肉，充皮肤，肥腠理，司关阖者也。

志意者，所以御精神，收魂魄，适寒温，和喜怒者也。

是故血和则经脉流行，荣覆阴阳，筋骨劲强，关节清利矣。

卫气和则分肉解利，皮肤调柔，腠理致密矣。

志意和则精神专直，魂魄不散，悔怒不起，五藏不受邪矣。

寒温和则六府化谷，风痹不作，经脉通利，支节得安矣。

此人之常平也。五藏者，所以藏精神血气魂魄者也。六府者，所以化水谷而行津液者也。"

The intake of food and the reduction of its energy is a major way for the body to obtain energy from the outside world. Foods in solid state enter the digestive tract and are gradually digested into microparticles which can penetrate the intestinal mucosas. This process is completed by the body's digestion and absorption system. The microparticles which enter the mouth and stomach before being absorbed by large and small intestines are called the essence of water – food which can be understood as tiny food particles. They are used by all the tissue cells of the body. Before the body uses them, it's required to finish a process of transformation and transportation which demand the participation of pulmonary respiration and blood. Thus, the effective perfusion of energy into a human body is not only related to digestion and absorption of food but also to respiration and blood transportation.

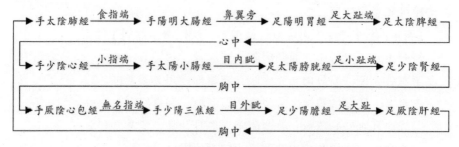

图 25 – 1　营气循行手足阴阳十二经详图

Modern physiological studies show that the emptying time of food by human stomach is 4 – 6 hours. That is to say, the process of food entering stomach, becoming chyme by the digestion of stomach, and then delivering to the intestine for further digestion and absorption, takes about four hours. This means that if a hungry person starts to eat now, it takes four hours for him to supplement energy and regain power. But it is not so exactly. Once one extremely hungry person is offered with a bowel of rice, he can feel the revival of power as soon as the food entering his stomach even though. It hasn't been filled up with enough food.

If a person is very thirsty after sweating sports, he needs to drink immediately. He would feel very refreshing and cool after drinking down a glass of cold water. But the problem comes, and he will feel thirsty very soon and needs to drink water continuously after that. Drinking cold water solves the thirsty feeling but ends up with drinking lots of water. The other case is to drink a little hot water. We all have the same feeling that drinking little hot water kills thirstiness and tiredness. Why? This is owing to the fact that human demand for energy covers both matter and driving force. The two aspects co – support physiological activities. This is the theory in Chinese medicine about how the water – food transforms into nutrient Qi and defensive Qi.

Five – zang temples and six – fu bowels system

From the discussion of past several chapters above, we already know that "Five – zang temples" is a virtual concept derived from an energy model. But human being is a tangible object which should have corresponding organs to accomplish the metabolism function of water – food. The six – fu bowels system of the human body implements the functions of digestion, absorption and transportation of food, and the five – zang temples system, containing heart, liver, spleen, lung, and kidney, completes the mediation function. The five – zang temples and six bowels constitute the human body system and are connected one another with meridians. The five – zang temples correspond to the anatomy of the heart, lung, liver, spleen and kidney, and the six – fu bowels correspond to the anatomy of the small and large intestines, the bile, stomach, bladder and triple energizers fascia.

营气与卫气

The generation of nutrient Qi

Food is decomposed to the essence of water – food by digestion which then enters to intramural vessel of small intestine and lymph gland through mucosal epithelium of the gastrointestinal tract. After converging step by step, the essence of water – food finally enters the heart though convergence by the vena cava and the thoracic duct, then transport upwards to the lung. From this, we can see that the tissue cells of body do not directly use the essence of water – food from the intestine tracts, which is transported to the heart first, then to the lung and finally chemically reacted with air in the lung. The process of turning food into the essence is completed by the participation of stomach, small intestine, large intestine, triple energizers fascia. The stomach is mainly responsible for receiving food and decomposition, the small intestine mainly for controlling the reception of digested food, the large intestine for transportation, the gall bladder for regulating, the bladder for gasifying fluid and the tri – jiao for regulating fluid passage. The essence of water – food is transported to the lungs by the cooperation of the six – fu bowels, and reacts with the air there to generate the nutrient Qi. By circulating it through the blood, the nutrient Qi diffuse into the whole body and is used by tissue cells. From this we can see that the quality of nutrient Qi is not only relevant to the food intake but also relevant to the quality and adequacy of air in the lungs.

Distinguishment and analysis of Nutrient Qi and Defensive Qi

With food entering the stomach, its energy would be finally divided into two parts: the clear Qi of nutrient Qi and the turbid Qi of defensive Qi. Since the turbid Qi has the characteristics of strong power and rapid flow, it can rapidly spread body and run the outside of meridian vessels and is called the defensive Qi. Thus, the defensive Qi can rapidly fill the human body. The difference between cold and hot water when drinking lies in the fact that the higher temperature increases the power of defensive Qi which can rapidly spread. Thus it has good effect of solving thirsty. The turbid Qi part in food can diffuse the body rapidly after entering the stomach. Thus, hot food and cooked food with pungent, fresh and fragrant tastes are more beneficial to human body. The characteristic of defensive Qi is to strengthen the functions of cells by themselves, nourish the viscera and bowels, protect the surface of the skin, open sweat pore and prevent external pathogens. In contrast, nutrient Qi is the nutritional ingredient of food. In a simple analogy, if we need to build a city, we need artisans as well as building materials. The defensive Qi is like artisan, and nutrient Qi is like building materials transported by railway. The nutrient Qi flows back into the blood vessels and is transported to the five – zang organs and six – fu bowels and then nourishes everywhere until feet and hands. Therefore, the nutrient Qi runs inside the vessels but the defensive Qi runs outside of vessels. This is the process of the digested food transforming into nutrient Qi and defensive Qi in human body and providing energy for all the cells and tissues. If the nutrient Qi and defensive Qi are inadequate, then the functions of five – zang viscera, resistivity against illness and even a person's spirit or will-power would be relatively weak. This is the relationship between nutrient Qi, defensive Qi and human life.

Since the powerful and rapid Qi is the source of defensive Qi, the food material with strong pungent odor can generate more defensive Qi, and sticky and greasy food can produce more nutrient Qi. Ginger and Chinese dates can be treated as two representatives of the Qi that generates the defensive Qi and nutrient Qi, respectively. More than this, all the condiments with strong odor can be considered as food materials which can increase the defensive Qi. The relation between the nutrient Qi and the defensive Qi is that of *Yin* and *Yang*. The balance between them can ensure health. Either weak nutrient Qi and strong defensive Qi or weak defensive Qi and strong nutrient Qi could lead to diseases. It reminds us that regardless of the diet nutrition or drug proportion, we need to pay attention to the coordination of nutrient Qi and defensive Qi. Too strong defensive Qi will exhaust the internal Qi, and too strong nutrient Qi will result in viscous running of the internal Qi. Therefore, it says in *Yellow Emperor's Classic of Medicine*, human can live longer if five – zang viscera are strong, blood runs harmoniously, muscles relax, skin condenses, nutrient Qi and defensive Qi runs normally, breath smoothly, essence of food is digested successfully by six – fu bowels, fluid and humor spread in all body.

营气与卫气

Operation laws of nutrient Qi and defensive Qi

The operation of defensive Qi basically complies with the law of running on Yang at daytime, and running on Yin at night when sleeping. This can be understood as the defensive Qi coming out when eyes are opened, and then people start to do things. The defensive Qi goes back inside when eyes are closed. The defensive Qi running on Yin means to go back to the kidney by the *Kidney Meridian of Foot* and then to heart, lung, liver and spleen, and finally return to the kidney. From this perspective, the nourishment and repair effect of defensive Qi on the viscera works when human sleep. This is the significance of sleeping. The five – zang temples system is nourished and adjusted in sleeping and this is why the person lack of sleep would get sick.

The surface skin is the frontline of the body's defense. The defensive Qi enters the inside of body during sleep, if a person sleeps without quilt, resulting in inadequate defensive Qi in the surface of skin, the wind – cold would enter the body and leading to catching cold.

The operation routine and time of the nutrient Qi is like this: at daybreak, it starts from the pulse point on the wrist of lung meridian, runs to large intestine meridian, and then to stomach meridian and spleen meridian, to heat meridian and small intestine meridian, to bladder meridian and kidney meridian, to pericardium meridian and triple energizer meridian, to gallbladder meridian and live meridian, finally back to the lung meridian. This routine goes to repeat itself.

The six – fu bowels transport and digest food to form the essence of water and food. The clear Qi of digested food and air in lungs generate the nutrient Qi which runs inside the vessels. The blood in vessels, as the carrier of nutrient Qi, transports the nutrition to nourish five – zang viscera and six – fu bowels, until feet and hands. It is the circulation channel for material nutrition. The nutrient Qi needs to penetrate vessel wall and infiltrate tissue space, and enters to cell through cell membrane so as to play the function of nourishing and be used by tissue cells. This process is called the microcirculation of human body.

The temporal operation of nutrient Qi reminds us that the opening of microcirculation is related to time and the intensity of microcirculation is related to the physiological function of tissue and defense repair. For example, from 7 am to 9 am, the nutrient Qi passes through the stomach meridian, which means that the tissues and organs belonging to the stomach meridian system at this time are in an active stage of microcirculation opening. This is the best hours in a day with the strongest digestive and absorptive capacity, which is similar to the fact that the sun shines the east window in the morning and then shines the west window in the afternoon, and thus the received sunlight would be different at the different times. The characteristic of the time operation of nutrient Qi would greatly enrich our minds, which leads to the method of keeping health and treatment of diseases relevant to time in Chinese Medicine. For example, when the nutrient Qi runs more rapidly in the liver meridian, and the microcirculation regulated by the liver meridian opens, at this time, the liver meridian has the most powerful functions of detoxifying and storing blood.

View of life structure by TCM

The function of six – fu bowels is to compose and transform food into the essence, and transport them into all parts of body. Meanwhile, the six – fu bowels excrete metabolic wastes of food. The essence of water – food transported by the six – fu bowels transforms into the nutrient Qi and the defensive Qi in heart and lung whose operative paths are the human meridians. Then, what are the functions of the five – zang temples? TCM doctors believe that the human life level has a physical level and a higher level of non – matter, and five – zang temples are in charge of human spirit and mind activitives.

As it is said in the *Yellow Emperor's Classic of Medicine*:

Human blood, qi, essence and spirit are matters that nourish the body and maintain life.

The meridian can make qi and blood flow and promote yin and yang to circulate, lubricate the sinew and bones, and keep the joints smooth.

The defensive qi can nourish muscles, skin and interstices, and is in charge of the normal opening and closing of the sweat pores.

Man's ideation and will can govern the essence and spirit, make the ethereal soul and the corporeal soul concentrated, enable the body to adapt to the climactic changes in the four seasons, and regulate the emotional changes as well.

Therefore, if the blood harmonizes and the meridian functions properly to promote yin and yang to circulate, the sinew and bones are strong and powerful and the joints are smooth.

If the defensive qi functions properly, it will lubricate the muscles, soften the skin, and make the interstices compact.

Harmonizing the ideation and will, will keep the essence and spirit concentrated, and make the mind quick, the ethereal soul and the corporeal soul work

营气与卫气

well rather than scatter aimlessly. Without the stimulation of the extreme emotions such as regret or anger, the five – zang temples function well and are immune to the illed qi.

If the body can make good regulations and adjustments to the climactic and dietary cold and warm, the transport and transformation functions of six – fu bowels will remain normal. When the source of blood and qi is adequate, the meridian works smoothly, and the body will not be attacked by the illed qi and suffer from the wind Bi disease. Also, the joints can function properly.

This is what the healthy body is like. The five – zang temples are the places that preserve essence, spirit, qi and blood while the six – fu bowels are the organs that transport and transform the essence of water and food, making the fluid and humor circulate.

八风与信息

Eight winds and information

事物除能量属性之外，还有信息属性。能量的运动可以用五行模型来表达，每一行代表了一个基本能量状态。为了认识事物的信息属性，古圣根据气候变化带来的天地物候之变，设计了八卦模型。

天地能量交汇并在水土的参与下，形成了第三种能量场，这个能量场孕育了万物生命，这个过程古人称之为"天地氤氲，万物化醇"。在有形世界里，生命以形、色、盛、衰等信息表现出来。因为信息是随四季而变化的，四季是能量变化所致，所以能量和信息一体二相，为同一事物的两个方面。

在古人的眼里，地表生态环境是天地气交而成，这个生态环境随四季能量的变化表现出不同的物候状态，物候以信息的方式表达出能量场。一年之中风向随季节呈规律性变化，从效果上看，好像是一年中不同的风向给大地带来了不同景象变化：东南风一到，万物复苏；西风刮起，万物萧条。风好象天地能量的使者，不同的风向带来了不同的信息，引起大地景象的变化。所以古人选用"风向"来代表万物的信息属性。

八风的来历

春气西行，夏气北行，秋气东行，冬气南行，古圣根据一年当中风向的不同，东西南北四正方向加上四个45度的偏角，把风分为八个方向，用八方来风来指代自然界八种基本信息特征。用坎离乾坤震兑巽艮代表自然界八种基本信息，称为"八卦"。八卦置于八个方位之中，即"八风八方"之法。八卦本质上就是水土合德之后地球表面的八种基本信息，所以万事万物的信息属性都可以用"八卦"来界定，这是古人为了认识信息场采用的一种数理模型。

九宫八风图

人体与外界环境进行能量信息交换，外界的能量信息场，会引动人体内部能量信息场，这是人体与外环境之间"同气相求、同频共振"的作用规律。信息在人体表现为思想情志和思维活动，思想情志影响气血运行，所以良好的环境可以保持健康，又可以通过改变外部环境的信息场来治疗疾病。

身体要维持一个良好的内在能量信息场，就要从能量和信息两个方面创造一个适宜的外环境。可以这么说，古典中医中所有的养生和治疗方法都是围绕这个原理而设计的。在中国传统的生命观念里，"气"为能量的运行，"灵"为信息的传递，所以古典中医可以说是建立在气灵学说上的医疗体系。因为万物皆有气灵属性，在完整的中医治疗体系中，万事万物都可以用于养生和治疗疾病，这是一个可以在不违背基本原理的基础上任意发挥、无限创新的医学模式。由此可见这是一个多么庞大和丰富的治疗体系。因为万事万物随时都影响着生命，那么万事万物都可以用来改善人体生命的运行。所以中医不仅仅是有病之后的治疗之法，更是一个保护生命使之不生病的智慧之学。

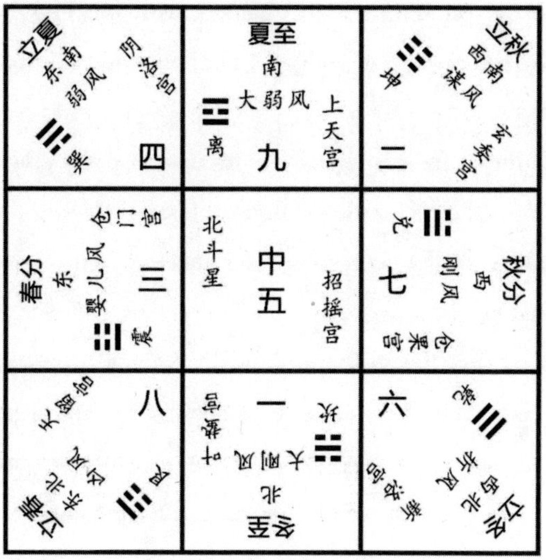

图 26 –1　九宫八风图

In addition to energy attribute, all things have the attribute of information. The operation of energy can be expressed with *five phases* model with each phase representing a basic energy status. In order to understand the information attribute of things, the ancient Sages designed *Ba Gua*(the *Eight Diagrams*) model based on the changes of world phenology caused by climate changes.

Under the circumstance of energy intersection between the sky and the earth with the participation of water and earth, it forms the third energy field which nurtures all species on the earth. Ancient Chinese call this process as "all species are born on the earth owing to the harmonious intercourse of the sky – Qi and the earth – Qi". In the tangible world, lives are manifested by information of shape, color, glory and decay. As information changes with the change of four seasons which are caused by the change of energy, the energy and information are thus two aspects of one thing.

For ancient Chinese, the ecological environment on the ground, formed by the convergence of sky – Qi and earth – Qi, manifests different phenological status with the energy change of the four seasons. Phenology expresses the energy field by means of information. In a year, the wind direction changes regularly with the four seasons. It seems that the different wind directions bring the changes of different scenes, that is, when the southeast wind arrives, all species revive; when west wind arrives, all species are bleak. Wind seems to be the messenger of energy of the universe with different winds bringing different information and causing the change of land scene. Thus, the ancient Chinese chose"wind direction"to represent the information attribute of all things.

The origin of Eight Winds

The spring wind goes westwards, the summer wind goes northwards, the autumn wind moves eastwards, and the winter wind moves southwards. Based on different wind directions in one year, the ancient Sages classified the wind into 8 directions by adding four included angles of 45^0 away from the four forward directions of east, west, south, and north, and they used the wind from 8 directions to refer to 8 basic information features about the nature. Eight Chinese characters,

Kan, Li, Qian, Kun, Zhen, Dui, Xun and *Gen* (The north, the south, the northwest, the southwest, the east, the west, the southeast and the northeast), are used to represent the eight basic information about the nature, called "Ba Gua" (*Eight Diagrams*). Placing Ba Gua along the 8 directions is the method of "Eight winds represent Eight directions". The nature of Ba Gua refers to the 8 kinds of basic information of the ground after the combined virtue of water and earth. Thus, the information attribute of all spcies on the earth can be defined with Ba Gua, which is a kind of mathematical model for the ancient Chinese to understand the information field.

Ninepalace Eightwind diagram

Since the human body exchanges the energy and information with the surrounding environment, the external energy and information field will trigger the internal energy and information field of body. This is the function law of "the same Qi absorbs each other and resonates with the same frequency" between the human body and the external environment. The information is manifested by thoughts, emotions and thinking activities of human. As thoughts and emotions affect the movement of Qi and blood, good environment can keep body healthy and we can treat diseases by changing the information field of the external environment.

For maintaining a good internal energy and information field, we need to create an appropriate external environment from the perspectives of both energy and information. It can be said that all the health preservations and treatment diseases methods in classic Chinese medicine are designed by this theory. In Chinese traditional life conception, "Qi" means the operation of energy and "Ling" means the exchange of information. Thus, the classic Chinese medicine can be called the medical system established based on the Qi – Ling theory. In the complete TCM treatment system, because all the species have the attributes of "Ling" and "qi", all of them can be used for health preservation and disease treatment. This is the medical mode by which we can practice using random and unlimited innovation without violating the basic principles. TCM is a very huge and rich treatment system because all the things in the world are impacting lives at any time, and thus all

八风与信息

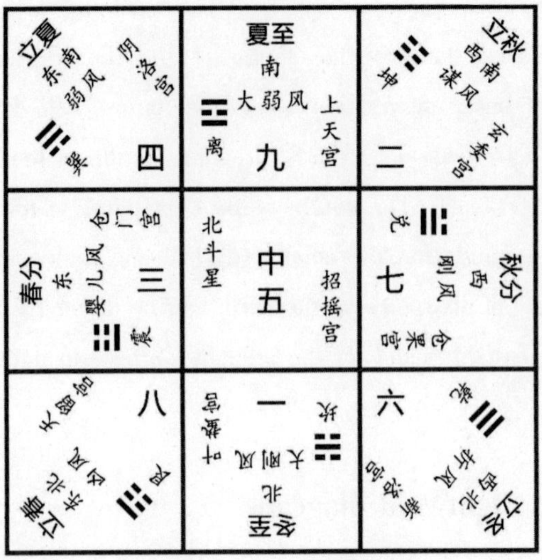

图 26 - 1　九宫八风图

the species on the earth can be used to improve the operation of human life. In summary, the traditional Chinese medicine is not only the treatment method after getting sick but also a wisdom of protecting life away from illness.